Feedback from Self-Practice/Self-Reflection (SP/SR) Participants

"As a professional I have worked with schema therapy [ST] for many years. Experiencing [ST SP/SR] has helped me with personal issues that other therapies hadn't reached before. It has broadened my overview of the therapeutic process. And it has deepened my understanding of the approach, values, and many elements of schema therapy. In all, [ST SP/SR] has expanded my capacity for being precise in my work. Thereby it has added to my professionalism as a therapist—so I can warmly recommend this to other therapists."
—SP/SR participant, Netherlands

"[SP/SR] was useful because it provided the space to think with others about the impact of the work. It felt like a safe space to do this because there were connections with others, but also the anonymity of not working together on a daily basis. I felt that the small-group self-reflections were most useful, as it was good to be able to use others' thinking and understanding of the modes in considering real issues. It is interesting that the same modes I struggle with in my work and personal life I want to avoid attending to (or I get stuck there) when I work with clients."
—SP/SR participant, Australia

"In ST terms, having had the experience of identifying underlying schemas, their activation, and the triggering of various modes as a client is extremely helpful to being able to connect with our clients and to understand some of their fear and even skepticism in engaging in experiential interventions."
—SP/SR participant, United Kingdom

"Reflecting upon my experience as the client in therapy, in addition to being helpful to my overall emotional functioning and well-being, gave me a felt understanding of some of my clients' experiences. I could genuinely encourage clients to allow themselves to grieve losses by crying as I could reassure them that they would stop at some point, allaying their stated fear that if they started crying, they would never stop. I could also say with authority that using a physical intervention to release anger a client was not entirely aware of could lead to some important information, as I had had the experience of being surprised at the depth of my own anger when I when I engaged in one of the self-practice exercises."
—SP/SR participant, United States

"I think that self-therapy is an integral part of education and that it is essential to the goal of knowing one's own triggers. This knowing allows me to be able to distinguish between my feelings (connected with my history) and the feelings of my patient, then to be able to come back to being attuned with where my patient is. It was a very important day for me and a great learning experience."
—SP/SR participant, Russia

"I have found it enriching and very helpful to have this experiential self-practice. Even though as a therapist you already have a cognitive understanding of the model and how it applies to you generally, I could feel that the SP/SR techniques work on a different level— one that I could not have reached cognitively. I will feel more comfortable doing this work with my patients now."
—SP/SR participant, Germany

EXPERIENCING SCHEMA THERAPY FROM THE INSIDE OUT

SELF-PRACTICE/SELF-REFLECTION GUIDES FOR PSYCHOTHERAPISTS

James Bennett-Levy, Series Editor

This series invites therapists to enhance their effectiveness "from the inside out" using self-practice/self-reflection (SP/SR). Books in the series lead therapists through a structured three-stage process of focusing on a personal or professional issue they want to change, practicing therapeutic techniques on themselves (self-practice), and reflecting on the experience (self-reflection). Research supports the unique benefits of SP/SR for providing insights and skills not readily available through more conventional training procedures. The approach is suitable for therapists at all levels of experience, from trainees to experienced supervisors. Series volumes have a large-size format for ease of use and feature reproducible worksheets and forms that purchasers can download and print. Initial releases cover cognitive-behavioral therapy, schema therapy, and compassion-focused therapy; future titles will cover acceptance and commitment therapy and other evidence-based treatments.

Experiencing CBT from the Inside Out:
A Self-Practice/Self-Reflection Workbook for Therapists
James Bennett-Levy, Richard Thwaites, Beverly Haarhoff,
and Helen Perry

Experiencing Schema Therapy from the Inside Out:
A Self-Practice/Self-Reflection Workbook for Therapists
Joan M. Farrell and Ida A. Shaw

Experiencing Compassion-Focused Therapy from the Inside Out:
A Self-Practice/Self-Reflection Workbook for Therapists
Russell L. Kolts, Tobyn Bell, James Bennett-Levy, and Chris Irons

Experiencing Schema Therapy from the Inside Out

A Self-Practice/Self-Reflection Workbook for Therapists

Joan M. Farrell
Ida A. Shaw

Foreword by
Wendy T. Behary and Jeffrey E. Young

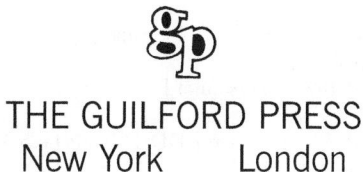

THE GUILFORD PRESS
New York   London

The authors have checked with sources believed to be reliable in their efforts to provide information
that is complete and generally in accord with the standards of practice that are accepted at the time of
publication. However, in view of the possibility of human error or changes in behavioral, mental health,
or medical sciences, neither the authors, nor the editor and publisher, nor any other party who has been
involved in the preparation or publication of this work warrants that the information contained herein
is in every respect accurate or complete, and they are not responsible for any errors or omissions or the
results obtained from the use of such information. Readers are encouraged to confirm the information
contained in this book with other sources.

Library of Congress Cataloging-in-Publication Data

Names: Farrell, Joan M., author. | Shaw, Ida A., author.
Title: Experiencing schema therapy from the inside out : a
    self-practice/self-reflection workbook for therapists / Joan M. Farrell
    and Ida A. Shaw.
Description: New York, NY : The Guilford Press, [2018] | Includes
    bibliographical references and index.
Identifiers: LCCN 2017055910 | ISBN 9781462533282 (pbk. : alk. paper) |
    ISBN 9781462535507 (hbk. : alk. paper)
Subjects: | MESH: Cognitive Therapy | Health Personnel | Self Care |
    Mindfulness | Practice (Psychology)
Classification: LCC RC489.C63 | NLM WM 425.5.C6 | DDC 616.89/1425—dc23
LC record available at *https://lccn.loc.gov/2017055910*

About the Authors

Joan M. Farrell, PhD, is Codirector of the Schema Therapy Institute Midwest–Indianapolis Center and Research Director of the Center for Borderline Personality Disorder Treatment and Research, Indiana University–Purdue University Indianapolis (IUPUI). She is Adjunct Professor of Psychology at IUPUI and served for 25 years as Clinical Professor in Psychiatry at Indiana University School of Medicine, where she developed and directed an inpatient schema therapy (ST) program for borderline personality disorder (BPD). Dr. Farrell is coprincipal investigator of an international study of ST for BPD underway in five countries and was principal investigator of a study of group ST for BPD, for which she was awarded a National Institute of Mental Health grant. A Certified Schema Therapist Trainer/Supervisor in individual and group ST, she is Coordinator for Training and Certification on the Executive Board of the International Society of Schema Therapy. Dr. Farrell is the codeveloper of group ST, with Ida A. Shaw, with whom she has worked since the 1980s. They provide ST training and self-practice/self-reflection workshops nationally and internationally and have written two prior books as well as numerous book chapters and research articles.

Ida A. Shaw, MA, is Codirector of the Schema Therapy Institute Midwest–Indianapolis Center and a Certified Schema Therapist Trainer/Supervisor in individual, group, and child/adolescent ST. She is Training Director of the Center for Borderline Personality Disorder Treatment and Research, IUPUI, and a member of the Training and Certification Advisory Board of the International Society of Schema Therapy. With a background in experiential psychotherapy and developmental psychology, Ms. Shaw is the main clinical supervisor of an international multisite trial of group ST and supervises the practice component of additional research projects on avoidant personality disorder, dissociative disorders, complex trauma, and child/adolescent treatment.

Series Editor's Note

Experiencing Schema Therapy from the Inside Out is the second book in The Guilford Press's Self-Practice/Self-Reflection Guides for Psychotherapists series. Research in a number of countries has shown that therapists who take the time to practice therapy techniques on themselves and reflect on their experience say that self-practice/self-reflection (SP/SR) has been one of the most meaningful and important parts of their professional development. These therapist observations are supported by a growing body of quantitative and qualitative evidence suggesting the value of SP/SR.

Once Guilford gave the green light to the SP/SR series, our thoughts turned to which therapies and which writers. Schema therapy (ST) immediately came to mind. ST has a coherent theory, well-developed practical strategies and applications, and a growing evidence base. Furthermore, ST places prime importance on the therapeutic relationship. For ST to be effective, schema therapists need to understand not only their own schemas (e.g., unrelenting standards, failure, and/or self-sacrifice) and how these may affect their role as therapist, but also how their schemas might mesh with or be reactive to client schemas. Therefore, a self-experiential and self-reflective approach to understanding one's own schemas is particularly valuable for schema therapists. Additionally, ST has important conceptual understandings and practical skills that may be learned and integrated better when they are experienced and embodied from the inside out.

Choosing whom we should approach to write the book was an easy task. I had already been fortunate enough to attend ST workshops run by Joan Farrell and Ida Shaw. Not only were their trainings highly self-experiential—exactly the orientation that was needed for an SP/SR book—but Joan and Ida had clearly immersed themselves in ST practices. They had no inhibitions about referring to their own schemas and how these interacted with their clients' schemas, and in spontaneous role plays they demonstrated an exemplary level of skill honed through many years of clinical experience. Joan and Ida walked the walk, and I was delighted when they jumped at the idea of writing this book.

For any budding schema therapist, this is a wonderful guidebook to learn the ropes. But, equally, for more experienced therapists, working through the modules will provide new insights and understandings, and new angles on therapy. Time and again we have found in our SP/SR research that experienced therapists seem to benefit just as much from SP/SR as novice therapists.

The fruits of Joan and Ida's professional and personal experience of many years have been poured into *Experiencing Schema Therapy from the Inside Out*. Drink well, and you will find that your skills as a schema therapist—and as a human being outside of the clinical context—will reach new levels of insight, integration, and intelligent application.

JAMES BENNETT-LEVY

Foreword

S chema therapy (ST) is an evidence-based approach that assesses the narrative linger-
ing beneath the client's self-defeating life patterns and carefully addresses the maladaptive modes and self-defeating patterns that emerge in the treatment room (Young,
Klosko, & Weishaar, 2003). Through integrated strategies from various bodies of work,
ST can effectively heal and reorganize biased beliefs and emotions informed by early
unmet needs and the temperamental makeup residing in memory and sensory systems
by replacing them with corrective and adaptive emotional experiences.

As therapists, we are not immune to the subjective and intersubjective reactions that
can emerge from our own early life experiences and schema-driven reactions to here-
and-now events. If left unexamined and unhealed, these life themes (early maladaptive
schemas) and coping modes can lead to frustration for both the client and therapist,
and poor treatment outcomes. The activation of emotional distress that emerges during
challenging moments in the treatment room can undermine the sturdiness of the most
competent therapist. In an attempt to regain stability and deal with the distractions
of tense and "stuck" feelings, we may find ourselves unawares on a familiar emotional
trajectory, where acutely reactive states trigger maladaptive coping modes—that is, giving in, avoiding, punishing, detaching, or defending ourselves with our clients. This
wonderful book provides a way to work through your own schemas in both personal and
professional contexts.

The Self-Practice/Self-Reflection Guides for Psychotherapists series, edited by
James Bennett-Levy, is a remarkably important contribution to the clinician's library,
with empirical validation of the benefits of practitioner self-work founded in cognitive-
behavioral therapy versions of self-practice/self-reflection. We are delighted that our

dear friends and colleagues Joan Farrell and Ida Shaw were invited to contribute to this invaluable series and have written this unequivocally instrumental book based on their global travels, research, and clinical and supervisory work with ST. Not only are these authors masterfully creative clinicians and implementers of research, they are also renowned international trainers with longstanding experience in effectively dealing with the challenges of difficult treatment populations, especially those with borderline personality disorder. The wide spectrum of vignettes in *Experiencing Schema Therapy from the Inside Out* is sure to resonate with the reader, as will the commonly shared burdens of our longstanding internalized messengers—ones that may promote shame and inadequacy; demand perfection, autonomy, stifled authenticity, and supreme sacrifice; or propose powerless surrendering to disconnection, mistrust, and the forfeiting of control.

With beautifully clear and articulate voices, thoughtfully relevant case examples, and elaborately helpful diagrams and illustrations, the authors show us how to apply strategies for schema mode identification and specific skills for forging awareness of our triggers while promoting healing of our emotional beliefs and responses.

Experiencing Schema Therapy from the Inside Out offers the therapist-reader an important guide for engaging the meaningful healing strategies that can lead to a reduction and weakening of defeating life patterns, while fortifying healthy and adaptive ones. We the therapists are offered an opportunity to adopt a firmer foothold when facing the challenges of disruptive moments in treatment and remain postured in our competent Healthy Adult modes, able to render the care necessary for effectively meeting the unmet needs of our clients—even our most challenging ones.

We are happy to share our support and to express our confidence in this book as a timeless and treasured resource.

WENDY T. BEHARY, LCSW
Founder and Clinical Director,
The Cognitive Therapy Center of New Jersey
and The New Jersey Institute of Schema Therapy

JEFFREY E. YOUNG, PHD
Founder and Clinical Director,
Schema Therapy Institute of New York

Acknowledgments

We are grateful for the invitation of James Bennett-Levy to write this volume, for his generosity in sharing reference material, and for his feedback on the manuscript version of this book. His assistance and support have been invaluable and led to a much better book. He paved the way for self-practice/self-reflection (SP/SR) in cognitive-behavioral therapy and laid an important foundation with his volume in this series. We would like to acknowledge the ongoing support from and opportunities for discussion of this work with Jeff Young, Wendy Behary, Paul Kasyanik, Gerhard Zarbock, Eckhard Roediger, Dave Edwards, Heather Fretwell, and Denise Davis. In addition, we thank Jeff and Wendy for their foreword and Eckhard, Dave, Heather, and Denise for their reviews. The Guilford Press's editors were patient and supportive throughout this process. We particularly want to thank Kitty Moore, Carolyn Graham, the very thorough copyeditor Margaret Ryan, and Editorial Project Manager Anna Brackett.

This book would not have been possible without the numerous therapists who participated in the SP/SR workshops we have offered around the world. We appreciate their feedback on this volume. Our supervisees have also taught us much in the course of our work with them.

We also acknowledge the support and love of our three little darling Yorkies, Ziggy, Zoe, and Zach, who sat under our laptops and in our laps as we labored through this bear of a book.

Contents

Purchasers of this book can download and print select handouts
and forms at *www.guilford.com/farrell-forms*
(see copyright page for details).

CHAPTER 1

Introducing *Experiencing Schema Therapy from the Inside Out*

Welcome to *Experiencing Schema Therapy from the Inside Out: A Self-Practice/Self-Reflection Workbook for Therapists*. This work is the result of many years of facilitating therapist groups with the goal of applying schema therapy (ST) to oneself and then reflecting on the process of that experience—what it means for you personally and what it means for you professionally in terms of understanding your clients' experiences and the ways you work with them. Both of us believe that the self-practice/self-reflection (SP/SR) process is an important, if not critical, component of psychotherapy training. The self-practice component is only half of the SP/SR experience. The other equally important component is self-reflection. The reflective questions move the SP/SR participant from personal experience to the professional implications. This is the difference between SP/SR and personal therapy, which focuses primarily on the personal experience. SP/SR is designed as a targeted, focused training strategy that makes an explicit link between the personal and the professional with a focus on both (Bennett-Levy, Thwaites, Haarhoff, & Perry 2015).

We have led 1-day ST SP/SR programs in ten countries over the last 10 years as part of the ST training we provide. Our belief in the benefits of SP/SR is based on our personal experience, feedback from psychotherapists in our trainings, as well as the research findings that support it (summarized in Bennett-Levy et al., 2015). We have both experienced a SP/SR-type group and personal individual therapy. We consider the self-practice of ST as a possibly ongoing, lifelong process. We feel that the work we did in our training years contributed to strengthening our Healthy modes and allowing us to stay grounded during the years that we worked with challenging and creative clients with severe personality disorders. The feedback from participating therapists, which is excerpted at the beginning of the book, has been very positive in terms of therapist self-awareness, understanding ST interventions, and in a better understanding of clients' experiences. As practicing psychotherapists and educators, the opportunity to write this volume and bring the experience of ST to an even larger group of therapists was very appealing to us. We know of no other SP/SR workbook using ST interventions.

In this chapter, we provide a brief introduction to SP/SR, discuss the rationale for including this component in ST training more specifically, briefly summarize the research evaluating SP/SR, and provide a "floor plan" of the rest of the book.

What Is SP/SR?

SP/SR is a training program for psychotherapists that combines guided self-practice with written self-reflection. It provides a structured experience of using ST interventions on yourself, followed by questions to assist your self-reflection. The self-reflective questions include reflection on your experience of the intervention, how you think this experience will affect your understanding of and work with clients, and how it affects your understanding of ST. The steps that we go through in the 20 modules of the program are essentially the same progression that we use in ST with clients. The difference in this therapist workbook, compared to our client workbooks, is that we provide some information on the "whys" of the interventions and directions on implementing them in your practice, while still holding the focus on your experience. For more information on ST and the implementation of ST interventions, see Farrell and Shaw (2012) and Farrell, Reiss, and Shaw (2014).

The Rationale for SP/SR

The workbook is designed to be of benefit to a wide range of therapists and students of psychology. You may be interested in learning more about ST, you may be at the beginning of training in ST, or you may be an experienced certified schema therapist and supervisor. Psychotherapists undergoing self-psychotherapy is a tradition that dates back to Freud. Traditional individual therapy focuses on the self of the therapist. The ability of the therapist to identify, reflect upon, and constructively utilize the content of his or her beliefs, assumptions, emotions, and behaviors, triggered by the interpersonal process of the therapeutic relationship, is seen as an important part of successful treatment outcome in cognitive therapy (Safran & Segal, 1996). Most psychotherapists who undertake training in ST have the experience of completing a self-assessment, including the Young Schema Questionnaire (YSQ) and the Schema Mode Inventory (SMI), which allow them to identify their early maladaptive schemas and schema modes. They also formulate their own ST case conceptualization using the same format as clients. Being able to recognize and respond to one's own schema activation and mode triggering when working with a client is a fundamental part of training and supervision in ST. Haarhoff (2006) identified the most common schemas found in therapists in training to be themes of unrelenting standards, entitlement, and self-sacrifice. She suggests that it is important in therapists' training and supervision to facilitate understanding about the potential therapy-interfering effects of these schemas being activated in work with clients. She speculated that the entitlement schema might be an overcompensation for the discomfort of the learner's position. Self-reflection is an essential part of ST supervision. The conscious understanding of one's own emotions, feelings, thoughts, and attitudes at the time of their occurrence and the ability to continuously follow and recognize them are among the most important abilities of both therapists and supervisors.

The importance of the self of the therapist is emphasized in the ST model. The ST model postulates that psychological problems in adulthood originate from deficits in core needs being met in childhood and adolescence. Consequently, gaps in emotional learning occur, which in cases of healthy development are filled by parents or early caregivers. In ST, unmet needs and developmental gaps (e.g., insecure attachment) are filled through corrective emotional experiences with the therapist (or group). For this reason, Young (Young, Klosko, & Weishaar, 2003) named the therapist style of ST "limited reparenting." In limited reparenting, a schema therapist must be able to be present and attuned to the client, and be a Good Parent who, within professional bounds, is warm, caring, and validating; supports emotional awareness and expression; sets limits when needed; and ultimately supports autonomy. These functions require a good deal of self-awareness in the therapist, comfort with his or her own and the client's emotions, and interpersonal skills. Self-therapy is encouraged and at times strongly recommended for psychotherapists in ST training. Therapists receive credit for these hours toward international certification as a schema therapist. A day of group ST self-practice is a required part of the certification process for group ST. In addition, dyadic or group role-play practice is a large component of ST training, which gives therapists another opportunity to experience the interventions, albeit by playing a client role. The focus on role play in the training of schema therapists is supported by the finding that therapists whose training includes a large amount of intervention practice have better treatment outcomes than those whose training is primarily didactic (Ten Napel-Schutz, Tineke, Bamelis, & Arntz, 2016). The self-reflection component employed here facilitates specific reflection on how your experience of self-practice affects both your understanding of your clients and your future practice with them. Thus, it goes beyond the focus on personal self-awareness of individual psychotherapy for therapists and specifically focuses the effects of SP/SR on professional practice. SP/SR has the potential to benefit both your personal and professional lives.

Research Findings: The Benefits of SP/SR for Psychotherapists

Our belief in the benefits of SP/SR from many years of leading workshops has been strengthened by the empirical validation provided by the research of Bennett-Levy and associates for the cognitive-behavioral therapy (CBT) version of these programs. The empirical validation of CBT SP/SR is thoroughly described in Bennett-Levy et al. (2015) and recent journal articles (Davis, Thwaites, Freeston, & Bennett-Levy, 2015; Haarhoff,

Thwaites, & Bennett-Levy, 2015; Farrand, Perry, & Linsley, 2010) We briefly summarize those findings here and refer you to the original publications for more detail.

The growing body of empirical research evaluating SP/SR for CBT demonstrates that the program enhances understanding of the model, CBT skills, confidence as a therapist, and belief in the model. Participants report "a deeper sense of knowing" the therapy. They also report enhanced reflective skills, a key metacognitive competency important for therapists' continued learning. SP/SR has also demonstrated changes in therapist attitude toward clients, with enhanced interpersonal skills and increased empathy for clients. Participants report insights and changes in the "personal self" and the "therapist self," enhanced reflective capacity, and use a more individualized approach to each client.

Through self-practice, therapists experience the difficulties of change that clients are asked to take on. There appear to be benefits for both novice and experienced practitioners. Psychotherapists with less experience report benefits in the area of declarative knowledge and intervention skills. Those with more experience report benefits in interpersonal skills, enhanced artistry, and metacompetencies such as flexibility and reflective capacity. There are even some therapist reports that SP/SR may also increase therapist resilience and decrease the propensity for burnout (Haarhoff, 2006). Bennett-Levy et al. (2015) suggest that SP/SR has the potential to play an important and unique role in therapist training and development because it integrates declarative understanding with procedural skills, integrates the conceptual with the interpersonal and technical, and enhances communication between the personal and therapist selves. Although as yet untested, it is reasonable to assume that the same effects would be found for ST SP/SR.

An Orientation to the Chapters and Modules of the Workbook

In **Chapter 2,** we provide a summary of the conceptual model and the interventions of ST. This is a helpful summary for those who have not completed ST training and a frame of reference for the workbook for those familiar with ST. We refer you to some of the key texts on the ST model for further study. We suggest *Schema Therapy: A Practitioner's Guide* (Young et al., 2003) for theory and *The Schema Therapy Clinician's Guide* (Farrell et al., 2014) and *Schema Therapy in Practice* (Arntz & Jacob, 2012) for interventions. For interest in treating specific disorders, we recommend *Disarming the Narcissist* (Behary, 2014) and *Group Schema Therapy for Borderline Personality Disorder* (Farrell & Shaw, 2012). *The Wiley–Blackwell Handbook of Schema Therapy* (van Vreeswijk, Broersen, & Nadort, 2012) is another excellent resource, with chapters on various areas of ST written by many of the leading ST experts.

Chapter 3 addresses you as a participant and provides suggestions about how to approach the workbook modules and the process of self-reflection. Therapists do not necessarily know how to reflect. This section contains a structure for self-reflection and suggestions for building your reflective skills. Self-care is also addressed, as this is still a neglected area in the training of therapists and one for which we think it is important to develop an individual plan. Taken together the first three chapters are designed to enhance your engagement with SP/SR and to support your efforts to derive the most benefit from *Experiencing Schema Therapy from the Inside Out*. **It is crucial to read Chapter 3** before beginning the modules, as it addresses the critical topic of developing a "safety plan" for yourself.

Chapter 4 describes the use of the workbook in a group format. We have presented SP/SR to groups of therapists ranging from psychology interns and psychiatry residents to experienced ST supervisors. For all, the experience is one that leads to both new self-awareness and increased awareness of their clients' experience in ST. The experience of one's Vulnerable Child mode being triggered in an exercise increases a therapist's understanding of the courage it takes for our clients to connect with this mode. Facilitating an SP/SR program is not that different for ST supervisors than ST group supervision, as ST supervisors must fill the roles of supervisor, mentor, and a therapist using limited reparenting. Facilitating a SP/SR group is different from leading a client group, but we have found that the reparenting stance—for example, stating that "you will be protected when in the Vulnerable Child mode"—is equally important for therapists and clients to hear. A key element in fostering engagement with the SP/SR process is ensuring that participants feel safe in sharing self-reflections. In Chapter 4 we discuss the guidelines that we have found useful for both SP/SR facilitators and participants.

The 20 modules of ST SP/SR are presented in six parts that are based roughly upon the phases of ST: bonding and safety, assessment and conceptualization, mode change work (divided into cognitive, experiential [emotion-focused], and behavioral pattern-breaking interventions), and autonomy. The progression of the modules mirrors the steps through which we proceed with clients. The modules are consecutive, and we suggest that you follow them in order as they build on each other. There are some important differences in this therapist workbook compared to our client workbooks. We provide information on the "whys" of the intervention and on implementing the interventions in "Notes" sections. Examples are given for each exercise based on three therapist examples, which we describe in Chapter 3, and there are self-reflective questions for each module. Since this is a self-practice workbook, another difference is that in Module 13 you will review the work you have done so far and decide whether to go forward with a deeper level of experiential work for the Child modes or skip to the Healthy mode work of Modules 19 and 20.

The Modules of the Workbook

Part I. Setting the Stage for Doing Self-Practice/Self-Reflection
Part II. Understanding Your Identified Problem Using Schema Therapy Concepts
Part III. Planning Change: Self-Monitoring, Problem Analysis, and Goals
Part IV. The Beginning of Change: Mode Awareness and Mode Management
Part V. Experiential Mode Change Work
Part VI. Maintaining and Strengthening Change

The Structure of the Workbook Modules

Module 1 provides some safety measures to use as you go through the workbook. These should be included in your personal safety plan, as described in Chapter 3. Module 2 has self-assessment questionnaires on quality of life and selected questions from the YSQ and the SMI. The remaining workbook modules are organized under the following sections:

- **Notes:** additional theoretical or clinical material for psychotherapists that put the module into the context of ST.
- **Example:** from one of the three therapists.
- **Exercise:** the self-practice section.
- **Self-Reflective Questions.**
- **Therapy Assignment** (not every module has this section).

Some of the modules have more than one exercise. You may decide to do one exercise per session and return the next time to the second exercise. Thus, you may spend a week on one of the modules, and 3 weeks on another that has more exercises. Go at your own pace. We suggest that you decide the number of hours you are willing to commit per week and then stick to it.

Your Engagement in SP/SR

Engagement in the SP/SR process is highly correlated with the level of benefit (Bennett-Levy & Lee, 2014). It is not surprising that engagement would affect benefit with SP/SR, just as it does for clients in ST. Some of the factors found to affect engagement include whether participation is mandatory (e.g., a requirement of a training program), optional (e.g., at the workplace but without any checks), and the amount of safety and protection of privacy provided. We suggest that if you decide to use the workbook, it means that you are able to commit some amount of regular, consistent time to it and to use the medium (self-led, in pairs, or group) that provides the safety and privacy that you need. It is something that you can do in stages, as we suggest in the evaluation of Module 13. It may be time to do some of the cognitive work, but not the emotion-focused or experiential work. Of course, keep in mind that to meet adherence requirements for ST, all three components must be integrated: cognitive, experiential, and behavioral pattern breaking. We expect that this work will make a difference in your personal life and therapist life just as it has for many therapists before you.

CHAPTER 2

The Conceptual Model
of Schema Therapy

In Chapter 1, we introduced you to the use of SP/SR for therapists, providing the rationale, potential benefits, and a summary of the research findings. The purpose of this chapter is to summarize the model, core concepts, stages, and interventions of ST that comprise the content of this workbook.

Background

ST grew out of efforts by Young and others to more effectively treat clients with personality disorders and those who fail to respond to, or relapse after, traditional cognitive therapy (Young, 1990; Young et al., 2003; Arntz, 1994; Farrell & Shaw, 1994, 2012; Farrell et al., 2014). Young developed the conceptual model of ST focused on individual therapy (Young et al., 2003).

At the same time, independently we developed a group model, initially focused on treating clients with borderline personality disorder (BPD) (Farrell & Shaw, 1994, 2012; Farrell et al., 2014; Zarbock, Rahn, Farrell & Shaw, 2011). We focused on developing experiential interventions to fill gaps in emotional learning and to provide corrective emotional experiences related to attachment and emotional regulation. Like Young, we used a limited reparenting therapist style expanded to meet a group's needs, including limited corrective family experiences. We moved from a focus on schemas to using Young's mode concept, and our model is recognized as a group version of ST. Recently, adaptations of ST for children and adolescents (Loose, Graf, & Zarbock, 2013; Romanova, Galimzyanova, & Kasyanik, 2014) and couples (Simone-DiFranscesco, Roediger, & Stevens, 2015) have been developed.

ST is a comprehensive, theoretically coherent model. Although ST strategically integrates interventions of other psychotherapy models, such as cognitive-behavioral, gestalt, and emotion-focused therapy, it remains unique. ST is consistent with the research of attachment theory, developmental psychology (e.g., Bowlby's attachment theory [summarized in Cassidy & Shaver, 1999]), and neurobiology (Siegel, 1999). One of the unique aspects of ST is its full integration of experiential, cognitive, and behavioral pattern-breaking interventions to accomplish the goals of treatment. All three types of intervention are necessary for adherence to the ST model. We speculate that the large treatment effect sizes for individual, group, and combination ST, described below, are due, in part, to this integrative approach that facilitates improved functioning as well as reduced symptoms and facilitates long-lasting personality change in clients.

The Empirical Validation of ST

The effectiveness of ST for clients with BPD has been validated empirically in several large-scale studies of individual ST: Giesen-Bloo et al., (2006); Nadort et al., 2009); one randomized controlled trial (RCT) of group ST (Farrell, Shaw, & Webber, 2009), and several pilot studies (Reiss, Lieb, Arntz, Shaw, & Farrell, 2014; Dickhaut & Arntz, 2014). ST has demonstrated effectiveness in a large multisite trial for Cluster C disorders (Bamelis, Evers, Spinhoven & Arntz,2014), a study of posttraumatic stress disorder (PTSD); Cockram, Drummond, & Lee, 2010), mixed personality disorder (Muste, Weertman, & Classen, 2009) and one for forensic clients with personality disorders (Bernstein et al., 2012). The effectiveness of ST reported in these studies includes improved function and quality of life as well as reductions in key symptoms and global severity of psychopathology.

These findings have led to growing use of ST and additional studies worldwide to evaluate its effectiveness with other disorders. Studies underway to research group and individual ST in combination include BPD (Wetzelaer et al., 2014), avoidant personality disorder and social phobia (Baljé et al., 2016), mixed personality disorders (Simpson, Skewes, van Vreeswijk, & Samson, 2015), and complex trauma (Younan, May, & Farrell, in press); studies of individual ST are underway for clients with depression (Renner, Arntz, Peeters, Lobbestael, & Huibers, 2016; Malogiannis et al., 2014), clients with geriatric issues (Videler, Rossi, Schoevaars, van der Feltz-Cornelis & van Alphen, 2014), and clients with dissociative identity disorder (Shaw, Farrell, Rijkeboer, Huntjens, & Arntz, 2015).

The ST treatment programs being evaluated vary in length from 20 sessions to a tapering schedule over 2 years and are conducted in a variety of levels of care (inpatient, day hospitals, weekly outpatient) and treatment settings (public and private hospitals, outpatient clinics, and forensic contexts).

ST is an approach that is rated positively by both clients and therapists (de Klerk, Abma, Bamelis, & Arntz, 2017; Spinhoven, Giesen-Bloo, van Dyck, Kooiman & Arntz, 2007). In addition, there is growing evidence for the cost effectiveness of ST in the individual modality (van Asselt et al., 2008; Bamelis et al., 2015).

Key ST Concepts

Core Childhood Needs

The ST model asserts that the etiology of difficulties in adult life lies in the extent to which the core developmental needs of childhood go unmet. These basic needs are for:

- Attachment
- Freedom to express, and validation of, emotions and needs
- Realistic limits to foster self-control
- Autonomy, competence, and identity
- Spontaneity and play

Figure 2.1 summarizes the etiology of psychopathology in the ST model.

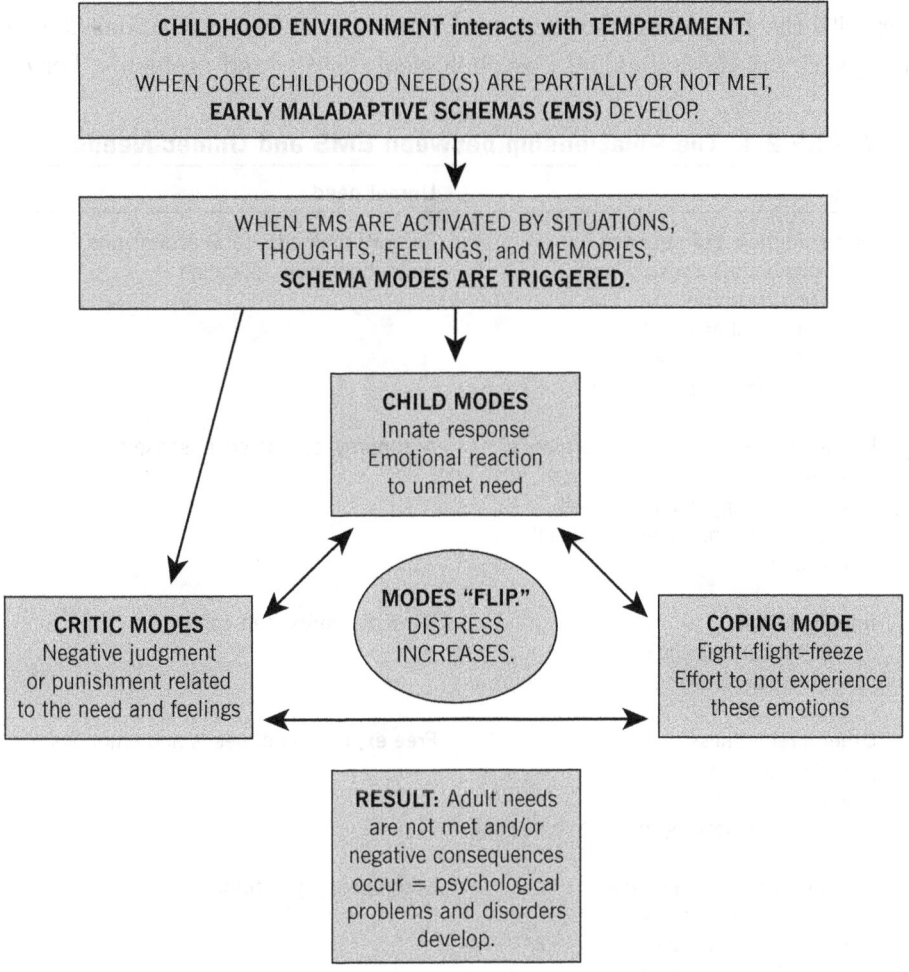

FIGURE 2.1. The etiology of psychological problems and disorders in ST concepts.

Early Maladaptive Schemas

The etiological model of ST assumes that when the normal, healthy developmental needs of childhood are not met, early maladaptive schemas (EMS) develop. EMS are psychological constructs that include unconditional and maladaptive beliefs about ourselves, the world, and other people. They are thought to result from the interactions of unmet core childhood needs, innate temperament, and early environment. Table 2.1 presents the 18 EMS that Young (Young et al., 2003) identified, organized around the five core childhood needs.

The ST definition of EMS includes memories, bodily sensations, emotions, and cognitions that are thought to originate in childhood and adolescence and are elaborated through a person's lifetime. They can filter incoming experiences and distort their meaning to confirm the EMS. These EMS often have an adaptive role in childhood (e.g., regarding survival in a depriving or abusive situation). However, by adulthood, they are inaccurate, dysfunctional, and limiting, although strongly held and frequently not in the person's conscious awareness. ST speculates that the number of EMS a person holds, together with the frequency, duration, and intensity of their activation, determine in part the severity of the individual's psychological distress and problems. For example,

TABLE 2.1. The Relationship between EMS and Unmet Needs

EMS	Unmet need
Disconnection and rejection • Abandonment/instability • Mistrust/abuse • Emotional deprivation • Defectiveness/shame • Social isolation/alienation	**Safe attachment:** care, acceptance, protection, love, validation
Impaired autonomy and performance • Dependence/incompetence • Vulnerability to harm/illness • Enmeshment/undeveloped self • Failure	**Autonomy,** competence, sense of identity
Impaired limits • Entitlement/grandiosity • Insufficient self-control/self-discipline	**Realistic limits,** self-control
Other directedness • Self-sacrifice • Subjugation • Approval seeking/recognition seeking	**Free expression** of needs and emotions
Overvigilance and inhibition • Negativity/pessimism • Emotional inhibition • Unrelenting standards • Punitiveness	**Spontaneity, playfulness**

on the YSQ, people with BPD endorse most of the 18 EMS at high levels of intensity (Young et al., 2003). Nonpatient populations (including therapists) endorse fewer EMS at lower levels that are activated less frequently. However, most people endorse at least some EMS. Similar to personality traits, EMS are always present but dormant until triggered. Table 2.2 presents the 10 EMS we will be working with in SP/SR, with their related unmet needs, typical childhood environments and their childhood and adult expressions.

Schema Modes

When maladaptive schemas are activated, intense states occur; Young (Young et al., 2003) terms these states "schema modes." **Schema modes are defined as the current emotional, cognitive, behavioral, and neurobiological states that a person experiences.** They reflect aspects of self that are not entirely integrated. Dysfunctional modes occur most frequently when multiple maladaptive schemas are activated. The four basic categories of modes—Innate Child modes, Dysfunctional Critic modes, Maladaptive Coping modes, and Healthy modes—are defined in Table 2.3.

The Maladaptive Schema Modes

The Innate Child Modes

The Innate Child modes involve the inborn reactions of a child when a core need(s) is not adequately met. These modes are often experienced as regressions into intense emotional states like the ones experienced in childhood when a core need, such as safety or secure attachment, was not met. In these modes, people appear much younger than their chronological ages and report feeling like a little child. Emotion is predominant in the experience of the Child modes.

The Vulnerable Child Mode

There are several variants and intensities of the Vulnerable Child mode: for example, Abandoned, Abused, Anxious, Lonely, Dependent, Humiliated. In ST, the variant a client experiences is identified and referred to with a personal name: for example, "Little Lonely Johnny," "Frightened Melissa." In the Vulnerable Child mode, a person experiences the distress of the unmet need with intense feelings such as fear, loneliness, anxiety, worthlessness, being unlovable, pessimism, and fragility. In this mode, a person feels the helplessness of a young child and looks to others for help and protection. This mode has many levels of intensity, from the awareness of a generally healthy person that his or her reaction is "too big" for the present situation and has touched a schema issue, to the desperation of a client with BPD who makes a suicide attempt to end the extreme pain of the Abandoned Child mode.

TABLE 2.2. The Development and Expression of the 10 Schemas We Explore in the Workbook Modules

Schema	Unmet need	Early environment	Childhood expression	Adult expression
Abandonment/instability	Safety, security	Unpredictable, lonely	Fear, clinginess, lack of connection	Others are perceived as unreliable
Emotional deprivation	Emotional support, empathy	Cold, withholding, detached	Lonely, empty	Emptiness, lack of connection
Defectiveness; shame	Acceptance, love	Rejecting	Insecure about comparisons, self-conscious	Hypersensitive to criticism; insecure, ashamed
Social isolation; alienation	Belonging	Isolated	Lonely, feels isolated	Lonely, feels isolated
Self-sacrifice	Child's needs are valued	Parents' needs come first	Others' needs more important	Acute sensitivity to others' needs
Approval or recognition seeking	Validation of self, uniqueness, and worth	Suppress self for approval; social status prioritized	Focus on approval, fitting in, at expense to developing self-identity	Life decisions inauthentic or unsatisfying
Emotional inhibition	Emotional support, validation; encouragement of emotional expression	Suppressive, rule-focused	Anger/aggression, play, joy, spontaneity are inhibited	Focus on rationality; difficulty expressing feelings
Unrelenting standards; hypercritical	Realistic standards	Demanding, perfectionistic, mistake-aversive	High standards, work to avoid criticism, little pleasure	Hypercritical, perfectionistic, rigid rules; impairs relationships
Failure	Encouragement, validation of strengths and abilities	Expectation of child's failure	Feels inadequate, inferior	Failure is inevitable, so why try?
Entitlement; grandiosity	Realistic limits	Sense of superiority	Special—can do whatever he or she wants	Feels superior, focus on power and control

Note. Adapted from Farrell and Shaw (2012).

TABLE 2.3. The Schema Modes

Innate Child modes	Vulnerable Child	Innate responses to unmet needs from childhood that are triggered in adulthood when schemas are activated
	Angry Child	
	Impulsive or Undisciplined Child	
Dysfunctional Critic modes	Punitive Critic	Selective internalization of negative aspects of childhood caregivers (parent, nanny, teacher, etc., adolescent peer group). Punitive Critic is harsh and punishing; Demanding Critic sets unreachable standards and expectations.
	Demanding Critic	
Maladaptive Coping modes	Overcompensator (Perfectionistic Overcontroller, Grandiosity, Bully–Attack, Approval Seeker)	Overused survival responses to unmet needs and trauma— variations of flight (Avoidance), fight (Overcompensation), and/or freeze (Surrender) triggered when schema(s) is activated
	Avoidant Protector (Detached Protector, Detached Self-Soother)	
	Compliant Surrenderer to any of the schemas; the person acts as if the EMS is true.	
Healthy modes	Happy Child	Modes in which adaptive functioning occurs, which is accompanied by a sense of well-being and fulfillment
	Healthy Adult	

The Angry Child Mode

The Angry Child mode is another innate reaction to not having a core need met, which may be vented in inappropriate ways, including intense anger, frustration, and/or impatience. The person feels enraged and may become demanding, controlling, abusive, or devaluing of others. An example is the tantrum of a young child when told "no" to a core need. In an adult, the Angry Child mode is characterized by a disproportionate intensity and a childlike form of anger. Often this mode flips to the Impulsive Child mode, and the person acts impulsively to meet his or her needs.

The Impulsive and Undisciplined Child Modes

These modes include selfish or uncontrolled behaviors when non-core-related needs cannot be met. In the extreme version of this mode, the person may seem reckless or manipulative to others. The Undisciplined Child has difficulty completing routine tasks; the adult in this mode postpones or gives up on boring work, monotonous tasks, or home responsibilities in favor of more enjoyable activities. These modes result from unmet needs and an absence of healthy limits in childhood.

The Dysfunctional Critic Modes

Young originally described these modes as "Parent" modes (Young et al., 2003). We refer to them as "Critic" modes because they also reflect the selective internalization of negative aspects of various attachment figures (e.g., parents, teachers, peers) during childhood and adolescence. The more general term "critic" rather than "parent" avoids triggering defensiveness and family loyalty conflicts as well as more easily engaging parents in the treatment of their children or adolescents. These two modes are experienced primarily via thoughts. A flip may occur to a Child mode and then the related emotions are experienced.

The Punitive Critic Mode

In this mode, a person feels that punishment is deserved; he or she blames self or others in thoughts or self-statements. When the messages of the Punitive Critic are verbalized, they become interpersonal actions and are identified as a Maladaptive Coping mode (e.g., the Bully–Attack mode). The Punitive Critic mode is a response to rules not being met, not to the *nature* of the rules, per se.

The Demanding Critic Mode

The Demanding Critic mode, however, focuses on the *nature* of the rules and believes there is a "right" way to do everything. In this mode, high standards are set and perfection is expected. Relentless pressure for high achievement is experienced. There is always more that can be accomplished.

Not infrequently, a combination of the two Critic modes is experienced.

The Maladaptive Coping Modes

"Maladaptive Coping modes" consist primarily of actions or behaviors and are defined as an overuse of survival-based coping styles: fight (Overcompensation), flight (Avoidance), and freeze (Surrender). All three coping styles have the goal of protecting the person from experiencing distress (e.g., sadness, anxiety, anger, fear). Because these modes usually operate outside of conscious awareness, a goal of ST is to help clients become aware of their use and to replace them with healthier, more adaptive responses so to get their needs met as adults. Maladaptive Coping modes are similar to the concept of defense mechanisms; these behaviors can explain the symptoms of personality disorder for both clinicians and clients. Three overall coping styles are categorized in ST as Overcompensation, Avoidance, and Surrender.

The Overcompensating Coping Style Modes

The Overcompensating style or "fight" contains modes in which a person acts in opposition to the schema or schemas that are triggered.

THE BULLY–ATTACK MODE

In this Overcompensating mode, the person tries to cause pain in another (verbally, emotionally, or physically) as a way to fight against a schema's activation (e.g., of Defectiveness/Shame). In its extreme version, the Bully–Attack mode can include antisocial or criminal acts and has a sadistic quality.

THE PERFECTIONISTIC OVERCONTROLLER MODE

In this mode, the focus is on protecting oneself from perceived or real threat by attempting to exercise extreme control over self and/or others. A suspicious version, characterized by vigilance, some degree of paranoia, and control of others, has also been identified.

THE SELF-AGGRANDIZER

The behavior of people in this mode is entitled, competitive, grandiose, and/or status-seeking to get whatever they want. They expect special treatment and believe they do not have to follow the rules of ordinary people. They act in self-glorifying ways to inflate their sense of worth and superiority.

THE ATTENTION/APPROVAL-SEEKING MODE

In this mode, a person always strives to be recognized as special and to get approval in an exaggerated way.

The Avoidant Coping Style Modes

The avoidant style ("flight") involves physical, psychological, or social withdrawal and avoidance to avoid distress or emotional pain.

THE DETACHED PROTECTOR MODE

In this Avoidant mode, a person is cut off from his or her needs and feelings. Although this mode appears to remove painful emotions, it is not a positive experience and it interferes with accessing information about what the person actually wants or needs. In this mode the person is physically present, but psychologically withdrawn. The degrees of detachment in this mode range from "spaciness" or a brief loss of focus in an interaction to severe dissociation. In the more extreme versions, a person feels numb, depressed, and empty. This mode is commonly present when clients enter therapy because it operates to protect a person in the Vulnerable Child mode from fear or the other painful feelings that may be triggered in talking about his or her problems with a therapist. Its forms range from a "good client" version in which a person is cooperative and superficial, not revealing emotional problems, to a robotic function. It is a common protective mode, and some amount of Detached Protector in some situations is a common experience even for healthier people.

THE DETACHED SELF-SOOTHER MODE

In this Avoidant Coping mode, a person shuts off emotion by engaging in activities that will distract him or her from feeling. These activities may be stimulating (e.g., work, videogames, random sex, gambling, dangerous sports, abuse of stimulant drugs) or soothing (e.g., overeating, watching TV for long periods, some computer games, oversleeping, abuse of sedating drugs). The main issue is that the activity is sufficiently distracting or soothing to allow the person to the uncomfortable emotional experience.

THE AVOIDANT PROTECTOR MODE

In this mode, a person is not present physically—for example, he or she avoids social activities, work, or any situation that is experienced as a threat that is likely to trigger strong emotions.

THE ANGRY PROTECTOR MODE

In this mode, a person attempts to protect him- or herself by putting up a wall of anger to keep others at a distance. Behavior is defensive, prickly, and off-putting—not to harm another but to keep him or her away. In this mode a person breaks the connection with others.

The Compliant Surrender Coping Style Modes

The third coping style ("freeze") represents giving in or giving up to the schema that has been activated. For example, if the triggering schema were Defectiveness/Shame, a person in the surrender response would accept that the schema messages are accurate—the person *is* defective and should feel ashamed, behave accordingly, never take on challenges, and work hard so as not to be exposed as incompetent. A person who surrenders to the Self-Sacrifice schema values and acts to meet others' needs before, or at the expense of, his or her own. The Compliant Surrenderer is passive, submissive, and seeks people and situations that maintain the self-defeating pattern of the schema.

Table 2.4 presents the relationship between modes and schemas in ST.

The Healthy Schema Modes

ST is a strengths-based approach. Two types of Healthy modes are identified in ST: the Healthy Adult mode and the Happy or Contented Child mode. Strengthening these modes to increase a client's ability to access them to get needs met in an adaptive manner is the goal of ST. The Healthy modes tend to be severely underdeveloped in clients with personality disorders. The concept of the Healthy Adult mode is similar to what Bennett-Levy et al. (2015) refer to as "New Ways of Being." In ST, there is a balance in emphasis between decreasing Maladaptive Coping modes and strengthening the Healthy Coping modes. The assessment of not only symptoms but also quality of life and healthy functioning in the ST outcome studies reflects this focus (e.g., Giesen-Bloo et al., 2006).

TABLE 2.4. The Relationship between Modes and Schemas

Mode	Related schema triggers
Vulnerable Child mode (abused, lonely, anxious, dependent) *Awareness of unmet childhood need; primarily an emotional experience*	**Disconnection and rejection EMS** • Abandonment/instability • Mistrust/abuse • Emotional deprivation • Defectiveness/shame • Social isolation/alienation **Impaired autonomy and performance EMS** • Dependence/incompetence • Enmeshment/undeveloped self • Vulnerability to harm or illness • Failure
Angry Child mode (impulsive, undisciplined) *Deficits in childhood guidance and teaching; primarily an emotional experience*	**Impaired limits EMS** • Insufficient self-control/self-discipline • Entitlement/grandiosity
Dysfunctional Critic modes (demanding, punitive) *The internalization of negative aspects of caregivers or significant figures in childhood and adolescence*	**Overvigilance and inhibition EMS** • Unrelenting standards/hypercriticalness • Punitiveness • Negativity/pessimism • Emotional inhibition
Maladaptive Coping modes (avoidant, overcompensation, compliant surrender) *Fight, flight or freeze responses to painful or negative emotion*	**Other-directedness EMS** • Approval seeking/recognition seeking • Self-sacrifice • Subjugation

The Healthy Adult Mode

This mode includes useful and adaptive thoughts and behaviors and the skills needed to function in adult life. This is the healthy, competent part of us that nurtures, validates, and affirms the Vulnerable Child mode; sets limits for the Angry and Impulsive Child modes; promotes and supports the Happy Child mode; combats and eventually replaces the Maladaptive Coping modes; and neutralizes or moderates the Dysfunctional Critic modes. The adult in this mode also performs appropriate functions such as working, parenting, acting responsibly, and committing to obligations; pursuing pleasurable adult activities such as intellectual, aesthetic, and cultural interests and hobbies; engaging in consensual sex; and enacting health maintenance routines such as ensuring a healthy diet and adequate exercise.

The Happy Child Mode

In the Happy Child mode, a person feels contented because core emotional needs are met. In this state a person can be playful, at ease, self-validated, connected, optimistic, and competent. Access to the Happy Child mode is necessary to engage in playful and enjoyable activities, particularly in social settings. Many clients were neither allowed nor encouraged to play, thus missing opportunities to explore their likes and dislikes and take part in the earliest form of social interactions. The Happy Child mode provides an important counterbalance to the pain of the Vulnerable Child mode. Experiences of pleasure and joy can keep motivation up for the hard work of ST and provide hope that life can be better.

Understanding Psychological Problems and Psychopathology in Mode Terms

Psychological disorders, symptoms, and problems in living of varying degrees of severity can all be described and understood in terms of the operation of schemas and modes. Mode concepts provide a user-friendly language for clients and clinicians and are our focus in the modules of the SP/SR workbook. Typical negative coping responses—aggression, hostility, manipulation, exploitation, dominance, recognition-seeking, stimulation-seeking, impulsivity, substance abuse, excessive compliance, overdependence, excessive self-reliance, compulsivity, inhibition, psychological withdrawal, social isolation, and situational and emotional avoidance—can all be understood in mode terms. Modes can switch rapidly in clients suffering from severe personality disorders, resulting in the sudden changes in behavior or seemingly disproportionate reactions that are one source of clients' interpersonal difficulties and emotional and behavioral instability. Figure 2.2 shows the three main patterns of mode flipping or switching. Modes can also stay rigidly entrenched, as is the case with many avoidant clients.

When schemas are activated, modes are triggered. Three patterns of triggering are possible, as shown below.		
Child mode → (**Emotion**)	Coping mode → (**Behavior**)	Another mode flip may or may not occur. The underlying need is not met or partially met or negative consequences occur.
Child mode → (**Emotion**)	Critic mode → (**Cognition**)	Coping mode → (**Behavior**)	Another mode flip may or may not occur. The underlying need is not met or partially met or negative consequences occur.
Critic mode → (**Cognition**)	Child mode → (**Emotion**)	Coping mode → (**Behavior**)	

FIGURE 2.2. Patterns of mode flipping.

The hypothesized mode conceptualizations of a variety of disorders have been empirically validated in two large-scale studies (Lobbestael, van Vreeswijk, & Arntz, 2008; Bamelis, Renner, Heidkamp, & Arntz, 2010). The main findings are summarized in Table 2.5. The modes of psychotherapists are included as well. To our knowledge, these modes have not been explored empirically, but are based upon our observation of hundreds of therapists in training.

TABLE 2.5. Mode Profiles by Group

	Child modes	Coping modes	Critic modes	Healthy modes
Borderline personality disorder	Abandoned, angry	Detached Protector, Bully Attack	Punitive	Few
Narcissistic personality disorder	Lonely, enraged	Self-Aggrandizer, Detached Self-Soother	Demanding	Healthy Adult (endorsed)
Antisocial personality disorder	Abused, abandoned, enraged	Bully–Attack conning or predator versions	Punitive	May endorse Healthy Adult, but little indication of it
Avoidant personality disorder	Lonely	Avoidant Protector, Detached Self-Soother	Punitive	Few
Dependent personality disorder	Dependent	Compliant Surrender	Punitive	Few
Obsessive–compulsive personality disorder	Lonely	Perfectionistic Overcontroller	Demanding	Some
Paranoid personality disorder	Humiliated, abused	Suspicious Overcontroller	Punitive	Few
Healthy psychotherapists	Vulnerable Child	Perfectionistic Overcontroller, Detached Protector, or Detached Self-Soother	Demanding	Present

The Goals of ST in Mode Terms

The overarching goal of ST is to develop the Healthy Adult mode so that a person can maintain a fulfilling life that includes work/career, obligations, commitments, satisfying relationships, healthy sex life, hobbies, recreation, and fun. When dysfunctional modes are triggered, this is the mode that needs to be accessed to perform the following functions:

- **Care for the Vulnerable Child mode.** This requires the presence of an internal "Good Parent" who can comfort and/or act to meet the underlying need when Vulnerable Child mode feelings of fear, sadness, or loneliness are triggered.
- **Become aware of and replace the Maladaptive Coping modes** with adaptive coping behavior that has little or no negative consequences—for example, be able to experience emotions when they arise, connect with others, and express needs. Active choices are made that meet needs and fit the reality of the adult situation the person is in, rather than defaulting to a Maladaptive Coping mode such as the Detached Protector.
- **Replace the behavior of the Angry or Impulsive/Undisciplined Child mode** with appropriate and effective ways to express emotions and needs (e.g., the ability to express needs and anger in an assertive adult manner). The long-term consequences of angry, impulsive, or undisciplined actions are considered.
- **Reduce the power and control of the Dysfunctional Critic modes.** Get rid of the punitive internalized critic, replacing it with the ability to motivate oneself in a healthy positive manner; accept one's mistakes and, when needed, make retribution for them, and moderate the Demanding Critic mode to have realistic expectations and standards.
- **Free the Happy Child mode** so that the person can explore the environment to learn about what provides joy in life and allows for play.

These are also the goals of the SP/SR workbook.

The Stages of Schema Therapy

The course of ST has usual stages with goals for each (Young et al., 2003). All three of the treatment stages must be addressed, but their order will vary based on the client's presenting problems, modes, needs, and the pace of each individual and therapist. This same order is followed in the modules of the workbook.

Bonding and Emotional Regulation

- Assessment, education, and understanding presenting problems in ST concepts
- Connecting with the Vulnerable Child (Safety)
- Getting around or through the Maladaptive Coping modes
- Affect regulation and coping skills (if needed)

Schema Mode Change

- Replacing Maladaptive Coping modes with adaptive choices
- Combating and challenging the Dysfunctional Critic modes
- Helping the Vulnerable Child mode heal through limited reparenting and corrective emotional experiences such as imagery rescripting
- Rechanneling the Angry and Impulsive Child into Healthy Adult action

Autonomy

- Development of the Healthy Adult mode and Happy Child mode and reliable access to these modes
- Individuation: following natural inclinations, pursuing activities that are pleasurable and fulfilling, accepting the responsibilities of adult roles
- Developing healthy relationships
- Gradual termination of psychotherapy with the option of future contact

ST Assessment

Questionnaires

The schemas and modes of ST are measured with two validated inventories, the YSQ (Young, 2017) and the SMI (Lobbestael, van Vreeswijk, Spinhoven, Schouten, & Arntz, 2010). Schemas are evaluated in terms of *intensity*, whereas modes are evaluated based upon their *frequency*. We utilize shortened forms of these questionnaires in Module 2 as your baseline measures.

The YSQ

The YSQ is a 90-item self-report inventory profiling 18 schemas. Each item is rated on a 6-point scale (from *"completely untrue of me"* to *"describes me perfectly"*). Evaluations in several countries indicate that the Young Schema Questionnaire 3 Short Form (YSQ-S3) is a sound instrument for measuring schemas, given its factorial validity and test–retest stability as well as convergent and discriminant validity (summarized in Bach, Lee, Mortensen, & Simonsen, 2015). The YSQ is available at *www.schematherapy.org*.

The SMI

The SMI (Lobbestael et al., 2010) is a 118-item self-report inventory profiling 14 modes. Each item is rated on a 6-point scale (from *"never or almost never"* to *"all of the time"*). The SMI has also been evaluated in many countries with consistent results supporting its factorial validity, internal consistency, construct validity, and ability to discriminate between subgroups (summarized in Sheffield & Waller, 2012; Bach et al., 2015).

Imagery

In ST, childhood memories of how needs were met are accessed through imagery exercises. We instruct clients to go back in imagery to an interaction with a parent in which a need was present (e.g., a need for comfort, safety, reassurance, or protection). We inquire as to what happened, how the child felt, if the need met was met, what action did the child take, etc. For clients with severe personality disorders, we do not use imagery for assessment until later in treatment, after a connection has been made and a safe place image established (summarized in Farrell & Shaw, 2012). We assume a strong-enough Healthy Adult mode in the therapists using this workbook to use imagery exercises to help to assess the origins of any maladaptive modes.

ST Case Conceptualization

The ST case conceptualization (in the context of self-practice, referred to as a "Self-Conceptualization") is a collaborative effort of client and therapist. The ST case conceptualization describes the joint understanding of therapist and client of how the current problems formed, the schemas and modes maintaining them, and the plan for ST treatment. The result of ongoing revision as understanding increases, the case conceptualization includes current major problems and life patterns, developmental origins, core childhood memories or images, core unmet needs, most relevant schemas, current schema triggers, schema modes, temperamental factors, and core cognitive distortions. A full conceptualization describes the therapy relationship, the impact of schemas and modes on in-session behavior, and the therapist's personal reaction to the client. Understanding the elements of a thorough conceptualization allows the therapist to choose interventions at any moment in time. A shortened version of the conceptualization is developed in Module 5. The full case conceptualization form can be found on the website of the International Society for Schema Therapy (ISSI; *www.schemasociety.org*).

The Interventions of ST

Limited Reparenting as Both Therapist Style and Intervention

Limited reparenting is both a therapist style and an intervention and is viewed as one of the active ingredients of mode change work. It provides corrective emotional experiences for the unmet needs of the Child modes, modeling of healthy action to replace Maladaptive Coping mode behavior, and challenges to the negative internalizations of the Dysfunctional Critic modes. The behaviors of the schema therapist during limited reparenting can be summed up as "doing what a Good Parent would do" in meeting the client's needs within the bounds of a professional therapy relationship. This means providing (1) protection, validation, and comfort for the Vulnerable Child mode; (2) the opportunity to vent and be heard for the Angry Child; and (3) empathic confrontation and limit setting for the Impulsive or Undisciplined Child mode. When working with the Vulnerable Child mode, we sound like parents talking to a young, frightened child. When confronted with Maladaptive Coping modes, we can become almost as firm as a drill sergeant—while at the same time letting the client know that we empathize with the feelings and needs underneath the mode. Active reparenting is needed early in treatment for clients with personality disorders or complex trauma, as clients are frequently in Child modes and have underdeveloped Healthy modes. Later, when there is more Healthy mode available, the therapist's role changes to being a "parent" of an adolescent and eventually of an adult. In this later phase of therapy clients still need connection with the therapist but can do most of their own "parenting" from what they have internalized into their Healthy Adult. The language, sophistication, and the use of specific ST techniques must be adapted to the developmental level, comorbid disorders, and psychological health of the client (i.e., some techniques and terminology that may be helpful for clients with BPD may not be acceptable to those with narcissistic personality disorder). When working with healthier clients who may have only infrequent triggering of the Vulnerable Child mode and a much stronger Healthy Adult mode, the reparenting style would be adjusted accordingly.

The goal of limited reparenting is to establish an active, supportive, and genuine relationship with the client that provides a safe environment in which the client feels safe enough to be vulnerable and to express emotions and needs. The therapist's provision of limited reparenting in the psychotherapy relationship fills critical gaps in emotional learning in the form of secure attachment and accurate mirroring, which leads to the client feeling valued and worthy, often for the first time. Initially, the therapist tries to compensate for the deficits in how childhood emotional needs were met within the limits of appropriate professional boundaries. Table 2.6 displays the limited reparenting response needed for each of the mode experiences and corresponding unmet needs of clients. The schema therapist initially assesses these needs and the strength of a client's Healthy Adult mode to choose an appropriate reparenting approach. An example could be the therapist's meeting of the need for soothing in a client with a severe emotional deprivation schema by draping a shawl around the client, wrapping it snugly,

TABLE 2.6. Mode–Need–Intervention (Ways to Meet Need)

Schema mode experience	Unmet childhood needs	Therapist intervention: limited reparenting
Vulnerable Child Experiences intense feelings of sadness, loneliness, and anxiety. Emotional pain and fear can become overwhelming and lead to flips into the Maladaptive Coping modes.	Secure attachment (includes safety, predictability, stable base, love, nurturance, attention, acceptance, praise, empathy, guidance, protection, validation).	Meet the listed needs by providing comfort, soothing, reassurance; wrap in blanket; connect with the Vulnerable Child in a concrete way to match developmental level. Listen, reassure, use soft tones.
Angry Child Vents anger directly in response to perceived unmet core needs or unfair treatment. Can take the form of a young child's tantrum.	Guidance, validation of feelings and needs, freedom to express, realistic limits, and for self-control.	Listen, encourage emotional expression, support venting, guide the client into safe anger expression (e.g., tug of war), set limits for safety or to prevent negative consequences. Help the client identify unmet needs to which he or she is responding; understand that the client may have difficulty thinking while very angry.
Impulsive/Undisciplined Child Acts impulsively based on immediate desires for pleasure, without regard to limits or others' needs.	Realistic limits and self-control, validation of feelings and needs, guidance.	Set gentle yet firm limits, provide guidance, and teach healthy release exercises. Help the client identify the need that is present.
Happy Child—this mode may be underdeveloped Feels loved, connected, content, satisfied.	Spontaneity and play, nurturance, attention, validation, acceptance, and encouragement to explore and play.	Take pleasure in the client and his or her playfulness and show this visually with smiles and laughter. Invite the client to play, and then play with him or her.
Punitive Critic Restricts, criticizes, and punishes self and others. Harsh, rejecting, makes all-or-none in judgments.	The Dysfunctional Critic modes suppress and reject the needs of the child—particularly the need for love, nurturance, praise, acceptance, guidance, validation, and emotional expression.	Stop the Dysfunctional Critic message; set limits on and eventually banish this mode. Support and connect with the needs of the Vulnerable Child.
Demanding Critic Sets high expectations and level of responsibility for self and sometimes others, pressures self or others to achieve them.		Challenge the message, reassess what comprises reasonable standards and expectations with the client. Support and connect with the needs of the Vulnerable Child.

(continued)

TABLE 2.6. (continued)

Schema mode experience	Unmet childhood needs	Therapist intervention: limited reparenting
Avoidant Protector Pushes others away, breaks connections, withdraws, isolates, physically avoids, uses detached self-soothing, dissociates. **Overcompensator** Coping style of counterattack and control. Do the opposite of the EMS. Sometimes semi-adaptive (e.g., Perfectionistic Overcontroller at work). **Compliant Surrenderer** Surrenders to the schema, acts as if it is true (e.g., if self-sacrifice, gives up own needs for others; if defectiveness shame, accepts self as without worth and does not try).	Any unmet childhood need can produce one of these Maladaptive Coping modes, and thus any need can underlie them. They are versions of the survival responses of flight, fight, and freeze and are overused and automatic. The immediate need is for connection and empathic confrontation. The long-term need is to learn healthy coping that fits better with adult life. That is the goal of therapy and requires developing the Healthy Adult mode. The Maladaptive Coping modes need to be reserved for emergencies.	Identify underlying need; for the Vulnerable Child, it is connection. Encourage emotional thawing. If angry Protector form, set limits and try to connect through it. Help the client identify underlying need and evaluate whether the overcompensating style is meeting it. Connect the client with his or her Vulnerable Child. Limit damage to group. Identify unmet need, evaluate whether coping mode meets it, help get need met. Connect with the Vulnerable Child.
Healthy Adult—this mode may be underdeveloped Meets a person's needs in a healthy and adult manner, fulfills the requirements of adult life, can enjoy life's pleasures, and form and maintain healthy relationships.	Acknowledgment and support of autonomy, competence, and sense of identity. Lack of childhood needs being met leads to underdevelopment of the Healthy Adult mode. The more unmet needs, the less Healthy Adult mode development.	Invite the use of competence, create opportunities to use and recognize strengths, and point them out with accurate positive feedback. Acknowledge and allow autonomy.

and verbalizing calming, Good Parent messages. These new experiences, interactions, and implicit attitudes that comprise limited reparenting become the building blocks for the client's Healthy Adult mode. Over time, the experience of the therapy relationship fosters clients' ability to care for their own needs in an effective manner and eventually to attain autonomy and healthy interpersonal functioning. This approach to needs is in sharp contrast to most other therapy models, which we see as focusing too early on trying to teach clients how to meet their own needs when they have never had the experience of those needs being met.

In the workbook, the therapist role is taken by the "Good Parent" part of the participant's Healthy Adult mode. Acting as your own Good Parent means being gentle with yourself when dealing with the experience of the Vulnerable Child mode, and being patient in evaluating the time it takes to accomplish changes in foundational aspects of yourself such as schemas and modes. Table 2.6 provides some examples of Good Parent behaviors in the column of "therapist behavior" to emulate in your self-practice.

The Three Main Components of ST Interventions

A defining aspect of all ST is the balance maintained between experiential or emotion-focused work, the cognitive processing of new awareness and insights from corrective emotional experiences, and the breaking of behavioral patterns. We find it helpful to divide the goals and interventions of ST into three main components, which are approached consecutively: mode awareness, mode management, and mode healing or experiential mode work. Clients (and therapists using the workbook) will need differing amounts of work in each component.

Mode Awareness

This component includes interventions that are primarily cognitive, with some experiential aspects. The goal is to teach clients to identify their own mode experiences, the triggering schemas, and the underlying need. Identifying the different aspects of experience—thought, feeling, physical sensations, and memories—helps clients become aware of the mode that is present. Connecting the current situation to childhood memories allows clients to understand the roots of their modes and schemas. Only after a client is aware of the mode he or she is currently in can the client make a conscious decision whether to stay in this mode or to access and use Healthy Adult mode skills.

Mode Management

These sessions use the client's newly developing mode awareness to plan for behavior change. Awareness is the first necessary, but not sufficient, step in the process of mode change. Next comes the evaluation with clients of the effectiveness of their mode-dominated responses in getting their needs met and forming and evaluating alternate action plans, referred to as "Mode Management Plans." Cognitive, behavioral, and experiential techniques are the primary interventions employed in developing and using Mode Management Plans. In this component, any barriers to change—for example, cognitive distortions, beliefs, or actions that maintain maladaptive mode behavior—are identified and challenged. The application of Mode Management Plans provides the needed behavioral pattern-breaking work that ensures that therapeutic changes generalize to behavior outside of the therapy setting.

Mode Healing: Experiential Mode Work

Experiential mode work includes visual imagery, imagery rescripting, mode dialogues, mode role plays, corrective emotional experiences in the therapy relationship, and creative work to symbolize positive experiences. To change modes at the emotional level, we develop "experiential antidotes" with clients. Clients often tell us, "I *know* in my head that I am not defective or abandoned, but I *feel* defective and abandoned." This statement summarizes the need to target the emotional level of modes, the implicational level of experience, to effect deeper-level change. *Knowing* that one is not defective or a failure does not eliminate *feeling* that one is defective and a failure. Feelings like these (implicit knowledge), with their accompanying shame, self-hatred, and fears of rejection, are what keep clients miserable, unhappy, and functioning below their abilities even when they have learned cognitive and behavioral skills. Creative and symbolizing work in the experiential mode sessions includes using art or written material that can facilitate recall and the emotional reexperiencing of schema-contradicting events.

Table 2.7 describes the goals by mode for these three components.

TABLE 2.7. The Goals of the Components of ST by Mode

Overview of the awareness component of ST: Primarily cognitive interventions

Mode awareness goals: Recognize your experience of the modes, learn to identify the beginning of a mode and eventually a choice point, and understand the link to childhood experiences.

Coping modes	Be able to identify in self; see as survival strategies from the past that do not get needs met now in a healthy way.
Dysfunctional Critic	Identify these messages, recognize them as faulty internalized negatives that are not accurate, and see them as "not me."
Vulnerable Child	Allow feelings of sadness, fear, and loneliness to occur without detaching. Understand these feelings as normal reactions to unmet childhood needs that get pulled into triggering situations.
Angry/ Impulsive Child	Recognize this angry mode in operation; see it as a response to unmet need. Learn to identify underlying need and the consequences of this mode.
Happy Child	Recognize and allow playfulness. Identify the modes that interfere with access to the Happy Child mode.
Healthy Adult	Recognize when you are in the Healthy Adult mode and be able to access it.

Overview of the mode management component of ST: Behavioral pattern-breaking interventions

Mode management goals: Recognize choice points and develop healthy actions to get needs met.

Coping modes	Be able to identify in self; see as survival strategies from the past that do not get needs met now in a healthy way.
Dysfunctional Critic	Have and use strategies to question and stop these messages and replace them with Good Parent messages.
Vulnerable Child	Allow therapist, as Good Parent, and group to meet the needs of the Vulnerable Child mode and be able to replicate their actions. Develop compassion for the Vulnerable Child mode.
Angry/ Impulsive Child	Identify underlying need and develop assertiveness, communication, and other skills to meet needs in healthy ways.

(continued)

TABLE 2.7. *(continued)*

Happy Child	Have a collection of playful images and commit some time to accessing this mode.
Healthy Adult	Be able to access this mode, develop and use skills to work on the goals of the Healthy Adult mode with other modes. Internalize the Healthy Adult mode of the therapist.

Overview of the mode healing component of ST: Experiential, emotion-focused interventions

Experiential mode work goals: Allow corrective emotional experiences in which needs are met through limited reparenting. These interventions are described in the Experiential Mode Change Modules 14 through 18 and Module 19.

Coping modes	Conduct mode role plays to demonstrate effects; use paper exercise.
Dysfunctional Critic	Use imagery rescripting, effigy work, critic jar, and mode role plays to banish or limit inner critics.
Vulnerable Child	Provide limited reparenting, imagery rescripting, and corrective emotional experiences.
Angry/ Impulsive Child	Allow venting of anger; demonstrate having fun with anger via limited reparenting.
Happy Child	Use play exercises and treasure box exercise.
Healthy Adult	Agent of rescripting, experiences of competence

The Need to Address Both the Implicational and Propositional Levels of Experience in Psychotherapy

Early approaches to changing EMS focused on content, that is, the propositional aspect of experience (Beck, 1976). Greenberg and Safran (1990) provided evidence that rational, language-based cognitive systems were independent of systems associated with emotion. It appeared that only implicational schemas were connected directly to the emotional systems, which means that they need to be activated and changed to accomplish significant change in the associated distressing emotions. Young, who trained with Beck, was instrumental in expanding the concept of a schema to include specifically addressing emotion and memories—the implicational aspect of experience—with emotion-focused interventions (e.g., adaptations of gestalt and experiential therapy interventions).

Our early work also addressed the need to address the emotional level of experience in working with clients with BPD (Farrell & Shaw, 1994). We were influenced by our clinical observations and the work of Lane and Schwartz (1987). They hypothesized "levels of emotional awareness" that are parallel to, but independent of, Piagetian levels of cognitive development, suggesting that these levels play an important role in the development of psychological disorders. We found low levels of emotional awareness in the clients with BPD whom we were treating. We developed experiential interventions to increase their emotional awareness and fill gaps in the early emotional learning that kept them stuck in extreme survival strategies that were ineffective in adult life (Farrell & Shaw, 1994). Lane and Schwartz view levels of emotional awareness as an important construct that is independent of diagnosis and can make a significant contribution to our understanding of the emotional level of psychopathology.

Bennett-Levy et al. (2015), in their CBT SP/SR workbook, also describe the need to address the explicit meaning, the propositional system, and the implicit meaning (i.e., the implicational system of experience). This awareness is built into the foundation of ST, and the emotion-focused interventions of ST were developed to address the implicational level of experience. The early integration of emotion-focused or experiential interventions with cognitive and behavioral pattern-breaking interventions is a central contribution of ST (Edwards & Arntz, 2012). The aspects of experience have also been described as channels: cognition, emotion, and behavior (Arntz & van Genderen, 2009). These three channels correlate well to the three types of maladaptive modes. The components and interventions of ST can be connected to channels and modes as a way to approach mode change work. Table 2.8 presents an overview of the relationships among mode, channel of experience, component of ST, and sample interventions.

The Foundation Program of ST

A detailed overview of the foundation program of ST, which combines 36 group ST sessions and 12 individual sessions, can be found in Farrell et al. (2014). This program covers the three main components of ST—mode awareness, mode management, and

TABLE 2.8. ST Interventions by Mode and Channel of Experience

Maladaptive mode type	Child	Critic	Coping
Channel of experience	Emotion	Cognition	Behavior
ST component	Mode healing; experiential work	Mode awareness	Mode management
Intervention examples	Limited reparenting, corrective emotional experiences related to unmet childhood needs, gaps in emotional learning filled, imagery work, imagery rescripting, mode dialogues, transitional objects, good-parent scripts, critic effigies	Education regarding your mode experiences, ability to identify mode triggering, ability to monitor mode, and ability to engage in cognitive distortion work	Access to the Healthy Adult mode is strengthened, with skills training provided as needed; plans are developed to meet needs with healthy action and refined through use.

experiential mode work—arranged by primary mode groups. There is a goal and a plan for each session based upon the component and mode of focus. Many of the self-practice exercises of this workbook are adapted from this program. For therapists new to ST, this program can serve as a general guide to working with clients. This is not to suggest that ST can follow a manual in the manner of a "cookbook." The mode a client is in and the relationship with the therapist(s) must always be considered. For example, when a client is in the Vulnerable Child mode, the priority of the therapist is to meet the need present in the moment, not to problem-solve.

Who Can Benefit from ST?

ST is an appropriate treatment choice for clients with personality disorders or features, chronic depression and anxiety, when other treatment has failed, when relapse has occurred, and for personal growth. ST can be described as "trans-diagnostic" (Farrell et al., 2014). As discussed in the earlier sections of this chapter, ST approaches treatment by targeting maladaptive schemas and schema modes rather than specific symptoms or disorders; thus, it transcends psychiatric diagnoses and changes in the diagnostic classification system. The presence of the maladaptive schemas and dysfunctional modes hypothesized for the various personality disorders has been validated empirically (e.g., Lobbestael et al., 2008; Bamelis et al., 2010). These concepts can explain the mechanism and symptoms of personality disorder, complex trauma, depression, and most anxiety disorders. Thus, maladaptive schemas and dysfunctional modes can take the place of symptoms as the targets of treatment. Modes can also explain less severe dysfunctional behavior found outside of psychiatric diagnoses in the lives of people (including psychotherapists) who function roughly within "normal" limits but experience "problems of daily living." Young refers to these as "stuck points" in his self-help book *Reinventing Your Life* (Young & Klosko, 1993).

ST can also be adapted to varying lengths of treatment. Three years of individual sessions demonstrated effectiveness in reducing BPD symptoms and improving quality of life (Giesen-Bloo et al., 2006), but so did 30 sessions of group ST added to nonspecialized treatment as usual (Farrell et al., 2009). Several studies are being conducted that test short treatment protocols (20 sessions or 4 weeks of intensive inpatient treatment) for a variety of disorders, with additional research in the development stage (summarized in Farrell & Shaw, 2016).

The Effects of Culture on ST

ST began in the United States and spread quickly to Europe and later Australia. It has the benefit of a strong international society, the ISST (*www.schematherapysociety.org*), which facilitates cross-cultural research to validate ST concepts such as schemas and modes and multisite international effectiveness trials. The issue of cultural effects on the development of EMS and modes is addressed in ST. EMS develop in response to unmet core childhood needs, which interact with temperament. Bronfenbrenner (1970) pointed out that the parent–child relationship does not exist in a social vacuum, but is embedded in the larger social structures of community, society, economics, and even politics. At this point in our understanding of such cultural effects, it is best to inquire about cultural influences as well as generation membership. For example, those of us brought up in the 1950s suffer the effects of Dr. Benjamin Spock advising our mothers to let us cry ourselves to sleep. When we are in the Vulnerable Child mode, expect the unmet need for soothing to be present.

Culture, of course, also affects psychotherapists. In giving trainings, we have observed many cultural differences in the way the core childhood needs are viewed and responded to. In Norway, as we demonstrated the validation aspect of limited reparent-ing for the Vulnerable Child mode, we were told, "We don't talk like that to children." Interestingly, those same therapists also commented on how good it felt to receive our validation. In contrast, in Greece therapists in training exercises could be effusive in their validation, but had more difficulty setting limits, another aspect of limited repar-enting. The Norwegian therapists seemed to have less difficulty than the Greeks in set-ting limits. Of course, these are just our observations of relatively small groups. Other cultural factors to consider in client assessment include religion and spirituality, ethnic and racial identity, socioeconomic status, sexual orientation, national origin, and gender.

Summary

In this chapter, we have summarized the main concepts of the ST model and described its goals, course, and interventions. The general goal of ST can be measured by decreases in the intensity, frequency, and inflexibility of maladaptive modes and underlying sche-mas. Modes provide user-friendly, understandable language for clients and provide the foci for psychotherapeutic intervention for therapists. Mode language focuses more on the role of learning and less on psychopathology, giving clients hope regarding change. We use the language of schemas and modes throughout the workbook. We begin the workbook portion here by asking you to identify your own schemas and modes. This is the process employed in ST treatment and training. The examples of our three thera-pists describe the modes and schemas that they become aware of through the assess-ment process and how modes guide treatment. Figure 2.3 presents a summary of the general course of ST. Table 2.9 is an example of the application of the model to "Julia," one of the three therapists whose examples illustrate the workbook. The modules also contain substantive "Notes" sections describing the concepts of the ST model related to the exercises.

BONDING
Safety is established. A safety image is developed. Connection is developed.
MODE AWARENESS
Awareness of a mode being triggered allows you to choose a healthy action that will meet your need, rather than allowing behavior from a dysfunctional mode to occur.
MODE MANAGEMENT PLAN
A plan for each dysfunctional mode is developed, which includes accessing your Healthy Adult mode and taking healthy action to meet the need that is present.
EXPERIENTIAL MODE WORK
Corrective emotional experiences are created that meet childhood needs and fill gaps in emotional development. These provide the basis for schema healing and the reduction of mode triggering.
RESULT: THE HEALTHY MODES ARE STRENGTHENED
You are able to meet adult needs in a healthy manner; your Healthy Adult and Happy Child modes are strengthened. Your quality of life and sense of well-being are improved.

FIGURE 2.3. The course of ST interventions.

TABLE 2.9. An Example of the Course of Schema–Mode Activation and Intervention

Situation	A colleague referred a client to me described as "challenging."		
Schema activated	Defectiveness/Shame		
Modes triggered	**1. Punitive Critic**	**2. Vulnerable Child**	**3. Avoidant Protector**
Aspect of experience	Cognitive	Emotional	Behavioral
Content	Message: "You are not good enough; don't even try or you will be discovered as a fraud."	Feelings of shame, fear	I usually avoid challenges and stay "under the radar."
Unmet childhood need	Validation of competence	Validation of worth and effort	Support for autonomy
ST component	**Mode Awareness**	**Mode Healing**	**Mode Management**
Intervention options	Provide education and self-monitoring; identify cognitive distortions, collect positive evidence, and reattribute cognitions.	Provide limited reparenting, develop an internal Good Parent; do imagery work, imagery rescripting, and mode dialogues.	Use empathic confrontation; develop pros and cons lists re change; develop plans to meet the need; provide skills training as needed; analyze results and refine plan.
Interventions utilized	Challenge distortions and all-or-none thinking, reevaluate childhood "failures."	Give myself validation and reassurance from the Good Parent of my Healthy Adult mode.	Made a pro and con list; decided to take on the challenge.
Was the need met?	Yes	Yes	Yes
Schema flashcard: to summarize the experience	"Even though I feel shame and fear that I am not competent, I know it is due to my childhood experiences and is not true today. For that reason, I will take the referral of a new client described as challenging. I will reassure my Vulnerable Child that my Healthy Adult knows what she is doing."		

CHAPTER 3

Guidance for Participants

This chapter is essential reading before beginning this SP/SR workbook. It will aid you in setting up your plan for approaching SP/SR, including developing a safety plan and aids for the process of self-reflection. The chapter is divided into five sections:

1. What you can expect from the program
2. The formats that can be used for SP/SR
3. Practical issues, safeguards, and good self-care
4. The process of self-reflection
5. An introduction to the three therapists whose examples are used to illustrate the 20 modules of SP/SR exercises

What Can You Expect from the ST SP/SR Program?

Experience Personal Growth and Increased Confidence as a Psychotherapist

Whether you are an experienced psychotherapist or still in training, you can expect to learn about yourself as a therapist and a person if you engage fully in the SP/SR process. In their studies of CBT trainees, Bennett-Levy and Lee (2014) report that the level of benefit from SP/SR varies considerably, from participants who said that the process is "life changing" and others who were unable to engage with it. In general, participants who engage well with the process report greater benefit, making it important to look at the factors that facilitate engagement. We expect this SP/SR work to help therapists become more comfortable with their own feelings, have increased confidence in using emotion-focused interventions, and be more comfortable with clients' strong emotional expressions. Bennett-Levy and Lee (2014) found an increase in confidence in trainees who completed a CBT SP/SR program. We expect the same effect for ST SP/SR. These speculations need to be tested empirically, as they have been for the CBT SP/SR program (summarized in Bennett-Levy et al., 2015).

If you are a schema therapist in training, we think that it is particularly important for you to experience via self-practice the emotion-focused interventions of ST, which you will be employing with your clients. The experiential component of ST is usually less familiar to therapists and the component about which they have the most anxiety when implementing. The majority of us were trained in primarily cognitive or cognitive-behavioral models, in which the inclusion of emotion-focused work is still relatively recent (e.g., Beck, 2011; Bennett-Levy et al., 2015). Others were first trained in a psychodynamic approach—either traditional or one of the newer versions (e.g., mentalization-based therapy; Bateman & Fonagy, 2016). When trained primarily in the latter approaches, therapists tend to be less familiar with the limited reparenting approach in which needs are met, and the active and directive interventions of the schema therapist. Experienced schema therapists may have somewhat different needs than beginners. Bennett-Levy and colleagues addressed this issue in a series of studies of experienced CBT therapists. They suggest that continued engagement in reflective practice supports the development of the competencies and metacompetencies important to supervisor and trainer roles. Research has demonstrated that SP/SR can result in a measurable change in self-rated CBT skills and empathy skills even in CBT therapists with an average of 18 years of professional experience (average of 9 years post-CBT training) (Davis et al., 2015). This impact was demonstrated at the level of both the "therapist self" and the "personal self." Participants rated their self-identified dysfunctional beliefs as significantly lower following SP/SR (Davis et al., 2015).

Accessing the Vulnerable Child mode in clients—the state in which uncomfortable feelings like sadness, fear, loneliness, etc., are experienced—is often unfamiliar to therapists beginning ST training, and it can feel uncomfortable and even overwhelming. However, it is important for you, if you are new to ST, to be comfortable with your own feelings and the experience of your Vulnerable Child mode first to be able to stay present to validate and sometimes contain the emotions of your clients. Anger is one of the emotions with which therapists are not always comfortable, nor are they at ease encouraging the venting those clients in the Angry Child mode need. To do ST, you must be able to meet your clients' needs for support of their emotional expressions. Emotional expression is one of the core childhood needs. It is one that many people seeking psychotherapy did not experience. Emotional inhibition and emotional deprivation are EMS common in clients and sometimes also in therapists. This workbook will help you identify the schemas that may be activated in you and the modes triggered in response to strong emotional expression. This awareness will help you to make a choice to stay present and not, for example, detach. In the workbook you will also learn how to access your Healthy Adult mode (particularly the Good Parent part of the Healthy Adult mode) when your dysfunctional modes are triggered in a client's therapy session.

Here is a personal example from Joan regarding a gap in her emotional learning, which she addressed with self-practice.

> Early in my work as a psychotherapist, I realized that I felt quite uncomfortable when clients expressed strong anger with raised voices. I grew up in a home where my mother was critical if anyone raised their voice, saying, "What will the neighbors think?" Consequently, there was little emotional expression, particularly of anger, even from my police lieutenant father. As I began exploring more emotionally expressive therapies, I decided to join a training group for therapists in which I could learn to deal with this discomfort and explore my feelings and triggers. After a number of sessions in which intense anger was being expressed and I hid behind a wall of pillows with some of the other therapist group members, I was able to stay present and eventually just allow the energy of someone else's anger to move through me without activating any schemas. The "hiding behind pillows" is an example of the Good Parent part of my Healthy Adult caring for my Vulnerable Child. Allowing that protection eventually led to the ability to access my Healthy Adult to work with clients' strong emotions.

Identify Memories of How Your Childhood Needs Were Not Completely Met

Imagery rescripting is an emotion-focused intervention that includes cognitive interventions in the postimagery debrief (e.g., cognitive reattribution, identification of distortions and evidence that contradicts negative core beliefs). This intervention is included in the workbook module on the Vulnerable Child mode. In these exercises, for example, you will be asked to go to a memory of a time in childhood when you needed a Good Parent, but no one was there. You are instructed to use a memory connected to one of the schemas you have identified as related to your identified problem for the workbook. (We strongly suggest that you *not* use a memory of significant trauma such as physical or sexual abuse.) You are then led through the steps of identifying the negative message about yourself or other people (i.e., the core belief) that resulted from that experience, followed by writing "what should have happened"—a scene in which a Good Parent is there to take care of the needs of your little child. After this is written, you are asked to construct this new experience in imagery and imagine it playing out with a "Good Parent." If you like, you can record the new experience in your own voice and play it back. This format provides an experience that is closer to doing imagery rescripting with a therapist. The final task is to create a new message based on this rescripted imagery experience. This is an exercise that is likely to create some temporary emotional discomfort, but it also has a resolution of those feelings and imagery work to facilitate positive feelings. In Module 13 you will go through a process of evaluating your progress in SP/SR and deciding about going further with the Vulnerable Child and experiential exercises or skipping to Modules 19 and 20 and wrapping up your SP/SR work.

Clients sometimes have some fear about, and a reluctance to engage in, the imagery rescripting intervention. Your comfort with the intervention and firsthand experience of it will allow you to have confidence and genuineness in encouraging your clients to try it, telling them what to expect, and even being able to say that you have experienced it. We think it is difficult to influence wary clients to "take a risk" when we have not done so. In SP/SR workshops we have had participant therapists do rescripting as a group with the same instructions as in the workbook. Many have used examples from their childhoods that were quite severe, but they still felt some relief at the end and a different message that contradicted their negative core beliefs related to the memory.

The approach of ST to childhood trauma is not to have a client reexperience it by telling in detail what happened, but rather to stop the recounting before something bad happened and create a new ending in imagery in which the child is protected by a Good Parent and his or her need is met. We do suggest that clients *not* begin with the worst thing that ever happened to them, but this admonition is not always successful. The closest we get to trauma in this workbook is to provide exercises in which you may experience the feelings that accompany memories of having a need and not having it met as a child.

Identify Some of Your EMS and Related Core Beliefs

Core beliefs are the result of the messages and rules that we take away from early experiences. Unlike some CBT approaches, ST asserts that addressing core beliefs related to EMS is an essential part of treatment. For this reason, they are included in the workbook. Nordahl, Holthe and Haugum (2005) demonstrated empirically the relationship between levels of EMS and personality pathology, and the ability of EMS modification to predict symptom relief by the end of treatment. In ST core beliefs are viewed as the cognitive aspect of EMS. Lessening the intensity and frequency of EMS activation is a focus of ST; consequently, working with core beliefs is an essential part of ST treatment.

You Can Expect to Experience Some Amount of Emotional Activation

To experience ST, you are likely to experience strong and, at times, uncomfortable emotions. ST is a "depth" approach that goes back to the childhood environment to identify the needs that were not met, which, combined with temperament, lead to the development of the EMS. When activated, EMS can trigger schema modes—a person's here-and-now emotional, cognitive, and physical state. Schema modes are the combination of an activated schema and a coping style. An activated Defectiveness/Shame schema combined with the Surrender Coping style (accepting the schema as truth) would lead to the triggering of the Vulnerable Child mode. In this mode, a client experiences some version of the shame, sense of worthlessness, being "wrong or bad" in some way that a child would feel when shamed and found unacceptable to a parent or caregiver. Of course, the focus in ST and in this workbook is to provide interventions that fulfill the unmet needs upon which these feelings are based. The client or therapist is not left in an uncomfortable emotional state. Experiential or emotion-focused interventions, which lead to corrective emotional experiences, are an essential component of ST, which integrates experiential, cognitive, and behavioral pattern-breaking interventions with the therapist approach of limited reparenting. We think that it is the inclusion of all four types of interventions that underlies the large positive treatment effect sizes ST is demonstrating (Giesen-Bloo et al., 2006; Farrell et al., 2009). Consequently, it stands to reason that part of this workbook would provide experiential exercises that activate emotion and the identification of EMS and related core beliefs.

ST has a somewhat different view of the role of emotion in the change process than that of traditional CBT approaches. ST can be described as the middle ground between the experiential therapies, which view emotion and its expression alone as adequate for change, and the CBT approaches, which focus on managing emotion primarily via cognitive skills. Attention to the emotional, cognitive, and behavioral aspects of experience and the use of specific therapeutic interventions to address them (experiential, cognitive, and behavioral pattern breaking) in ST provide all the needed ingredients for deeper-level change.

Is There a Potential for Difficult or Negative Experiences from the Workbook Exercises?

In using the workbook, you may become aware of a schema or mode that could benefit from some personal therapy. It is highly unlikely that doing the experiential exercises contained in this workbook will cause emotional harm to therapist participants. That said, the work may be difficult at times, and a minority of participants may have an uncomfortable or even negative experience with an exercise. Therefore, we empathize developing and using a personal safety plan for therapists just as we do for our clients. Clients often experience the emotion-focused work of ST as "different" from other therapies they have done. They sometimes experience it also as challenging at times and even scary. We tell them that ST may be the most challenging therapy they will do, but it can also be the therapy that makes the biggest difference in their lives. We reassure them that the coping modes that allowed them to survive trauma or unmet childhood needs will still operate to protect them in SP/SR. We also offer you this reassurance. The concept of Maladaptive Coping modes in ST suggests that if the emotion is too intense, the person's characteristic protective response (Avoidance, Overcompensation, or Surrender) will be triggered to diminish the emotion by flight, fight, or freeze. As they do for our clients, these default coping strategies will act as a limiting factor to your emotional distress. If you find that coping modes are being triggered frequently as you do the SP/SR exercises, the message to you is to look at the schema(s) involved, identify the leftover childhood need and the current adult need related to it, look at how you can meet this need, and go more slowly. This would also be a circumstance for which you might consider personal therapy.

Formats for SP/SR

Using the SP/SR Workbook Self-Guided

You may want to engage with the program in the workbook on your own due to geographical or professional isolation, a personal preference for privacy, or awareness that you do better on your own. If you choose to work alone, it would be important to set up a structure to support your doing this SP/SR work. One helpful structure is to set a regular time aside and schedule it into your week. When working alone, having a safety plan is even more important in case you have an unexpected intense emotional response to an exercise. This issue is discussed in the section on safeguards below.

Using the SP/SR Workbook with a Colleague

Bennett-Levy et al. (2015) report that participants in their SP/SR work describe benefits from doing the exercises and sharing reflections with a colleague—as a "buddy." This sort of interaction can expand self-reflection, provide support and encouragement, and add another level of safety. Obviously, there would need to be a high level of trust between the partners. You may also want to consider choosing a partner with a comparable level of ST experience and stage of professional development. We suggest that therapists new to the ST model choose a problem for the workbook exercises related to their work as therapists. For the more experienced schema therapist, a focus on a problem in your personal life is suggested. A pair with a shared type of focus is preferable. It is also important to share the discussion time equally and to avoid a partnership in which one takes more of a therapist role.

Using the SP/SR Workbook in Groups

As we have found in clinical ST groups, the therapeutic factors of working groups may amplify the effects of therapist SP/SR work. We frequently observe that one participant's sharing seems to elicit the sharing of another and that this interactive process continues. It is as if one self-reflection triggers another, and the interactive process amplifies or catalyzes the energy, leading to additional insights and emotion activating experiences. Therapeutic factors such as universality and social learning can add to self-reflective work and increase engagement. The support and validation of a group, together with the sense of belonging, may also increase motivation and engagement in the process. However, the type of group may affect the experience. Many types of groups can engage in SP/SR: for example, training-associated groups, those in workplaces, peer supervision formats, university degree programs, and virtual groups sharing a blog. The type of group can be expected to affect the amount of safety and confidentiality a participant will experience and consequently how much personal material is shared. Hierarchical groups in the workplace may be inhibiting for those on either the high or low end of the status ladder. When we work with such configurations, we allow the large group to choose how to divide into smaller groups based on participants' comfort level with their coworkers. This method does not completely remove the effects of hierarchy, but it seems to help with safety level. We also ask everyone in the group to commit to confidentiality for any personal material shared, and we do this openly, asking every person to raise his or her hand if he or she agrees. The SP/SR ST groups we facilitate are discussed in Chapter 4.

Using the SP/SR Workbook in Supervision

In ST supervision (as it is defined by the ISST, the certification authority for schema therapists) the effect of the person of the therapist on the therapeutic work is a major focus. We regularly examine which schemas were activated and modes triggered, and how to access the therapist's Healthy Adult mode. Discussing your SP/SR work in supervision would be consistent with the supervisory style of ST. You could undertake regular supervisory sessions for this purpose in the same manner that personal therapy sessions could be utilized. Whether review of SP/SR work would be the sole purpose of a supervisory agreement or used only occasionally is up to the supervisor and supervisee. Flexibility to meet the need present is a hallmark of ST, so many options should be possible with an ST supervisor.

In summary, there are pros and cons for the various options of SP/SR work, which you should evaluate based on your needs and the options available to you.

Practical Issues

Safeguards

Given the importance of experiential or emotion-focused work in ST, we are careful to build in safeguards for participants in SP/SR so that they can do the experiential work of the workbook safely and without undue anxiety about the outcome. One aspect of safety is to consider carefully the timing of doing this work. We think it is helpful to do this work while training in ST; however, if you are experiencing a period of personal instability (e.g., after a breakup, significant loss, death) it may not be a good time to use this workbook alone. On the other hand, if you are continuing to work as a therapist during such a period, SP/SR could be particularly useful in helping you to identify your activated schemas, triggered modes, and underlying needs. It is important for you to evaluate the effect of the workbook on your psychological health in an ongoing manner. ST views uncomfortable or distressing emotions that arise during exercises with clients as opportunities for healing. Schema therapists monitor client distress and implement safety measures and corrective emotional experiences. SP/SR, in its individual form, has no therapist to meet the needs or provide support around uncomfortable feelings that may occur. For that reason, we have added safeguards and the overall suggestion that you **stop if you feel overwhelmed,** take a break, and use one of the following:

Example: My SP/SR Safeguard Plan

- My Safe-Place Image (developed in Module 1)
- My emergency plans
- Exercises to access my Healthy Adult mode (Modules 12 and 20)
- Connection to a support system (e.g., the Google group overseen by us)
- Consulting a professional therapist or supervisor

Bennett-Levy et al. (2001) report that in their studies, CBT trainees occasionally have reported distressing emotional experiences when engaging in SP/SR, leading them to emphasize the need for safeguard strategies, including temporarily or permanently opting out. If you keep getting stuck in intense uncomfortable emotions using the ST SP/SR exercises, you may need to get help from a peer support group, supervisor, or therapist until you are able to regain balance. This is in no way a failure; it points out what may be an early gap in your emotional learning or an experience of unmet childhood needs. ST is designed to fill these gaps—for therapists as well as for clients. Awareness of being stuck can be used as a signal that you need to examine the schema-activated and mode-triggered unmet need—the path to overcoming your "stuckness."

Support for Your Self-Care Plan

Therapist self-care is an important topic that is frequently neglected. The Self-Sacrifice schema is one often found in therapists (Haarhoff, 2006). Just as we teach our clients to identify their needs and learn to meet them in a healthy and effective manner, we as therapists must do the same. The SP/SR program is helpful with this undertaking, and at times personal therapy may be needed for additional self-care support. The core of ST is a focus on needs being met. Reflect on your needs vis-à-vis this process. If you feel it is not the time to work on a particular module—don't. Use the time to take care of your current needs instead. Be on the lookout for negative messages from the Critic modes. They are not helpful to this process and have no place in it—kick them out. Do not expect perfection; it is not attainable. The self-practice exercises may lead you to identify EMS or Maladaptive Coping modes of which you were not aware. You may see how they affect your clinical work and begin to question your ability as a therapist. It is important to realize that through this process, you can become a more effective and empathic therapist. If therapists had to be paragons of emotional health, we would be a very small group.

Preventing Burnout

For all of us entering one of the "helping professions" with hope and enthusiasm, it is essential to remember that we must attend to our own well-being and preventive maintenance of self in order keep up the demanding task of providing significant emotional support of wounded others. The literature on the topic of self-care for psychotherapists is rapidly growing (Perris, Fretwell, & Shaw, 2012). In general, the term "burnout" is used to describe states of emotional exhaustion, depersonalization, and reduced sense of personal accomplishment in caregivers. Burnout is associated with a lack of close emotional involvement and inadequate support by peers, friends, or family. Additional risk factors include a highly empathic approach to therapy, working with patients with trauma histories, and having a history of personal trauma.

The first two risk factors apply particularly to the ST model with its focus on empathy, meeting clients' needs with limited reparenting, maintaining a high level of connection and transparency, and being genuinely present in sessions; and by the high prevalence of trauma in the client population for which ST is utilized, particularly the population with borderline personality disorder. ST focuses on core emotional needs through cognitive, experiential, and behavioral strategies, while relying on the process of healing within the therapeutic relationship. Therefore, to be genuine as schema therapists and have the ongoing energy for the work involved in limited reparenting, we need to be aware of and take our own emotional needs seriously. One important part of taking care of oneself as a therapist is emotional awareness and acceptance of one's own emotional needs.

Therapist self-care involves conscientiously attending to getting your own core emotional needs met and to those times when your Vulnerable Child mode is triggered. Of course, our needs should not be met by our clients or at the expense of meeting their needs. For example, sadness over needs not being met in childhood being expressed by clients can activate our schemas related to these experiences and possibly trigger our Vulnerable Child modes. If you become aware of your Vulnerable Child mode being triggered while in a session, you must find a way to acknowledge your Vulnerable Child mode's need, postpone meeting it, and then access your Healthy Adult mode to continue the session. Acknowledging your Vulnerable Child mode may be as simple as saying to yourself "I am aware of your sadness and need for comfort, and I promise to come back to you later today to meet your need." It is then crucial to find some time that day to reflect on the need present in your Vulnerable Child mode and act to meet it. This issue is discussed in Module 20 with the exercise "Walking through My Modes."

Some examples of good self-care include making sure that needs such as love, nurturance, and support in intimate relationships are met, and that you have someone with whom to share difficult experiences so that you feel guided, supported, and well connected while also retaining a sense of autonomy and independence. As is defined in ST, relationship and connectedness are core elements of well-being.

Attention to Your Core Needs

ST is an approach focused on core needs. In our clients these needs have often remained unmet since childhood (e.g., the need for an attachment figure that provides adaptive relational qualities such as nurturance, love, validation, autonomy, and empathic limits), which has prevented them from achieving healthy emotional maturation and growth. In ST, we meet our clients' needs within professional boundaries as part of the therapeutic style of ST: limited reparenting. The model asserts that the corrective emotional experiences provided by limited reparenting are a critical intervention of ST, particularly with clients who have personality disorders. Successful limited reparenting is thought to largely depend on therapists' interpersonal skills, such as emotional awareness and the ability to adaptively respond to core needs in the here and now in the therapeutic process.

Like all humans, schema therapists have individual limitations (e.g., issues of unrelenting standards, defectiveness, self-sacrifice) that can interfere with the practice of limited reparenting. Considering its personal and intimate nature, working within the limited reparenting model is more likely to trigger the therapist's own schemas and dysfunctional coping modes than more cognitive and behavioral approaches. Supervisory experience suggests that having our own schemas activated and modes triggered is inevitable. Schema therapist self-care—that is, attending to one's own needs—gives us the possibility to prevent or lower the occurrence of ineffective limited reparenting and to also increase our professional and personal well-being. Examples of some of the ways therapists can attend to their core emotional needs are given in Table 3.1.

TABLE 3.1. Examples of How You Can Attend to Your Core Emotional Needs as a Schema Therapist

Connection	Autonomy	Competence	Healthy limits	Spontaneity, fun
• Nurture your intimate connections (family, partner, and friends). • Express emotions, vent in safe places, and share private thoughts and concerns. • Maintain an ongoing, compassionate inner dialogue with your own Vulnerable Child.	• Nurture your core values in day-to-day actions. • Make choices that are self-aware. Find outlets for your own creativity. • Pursue your interests unrelated to psychotherapy— e.g., travel, hobbies.	• Take workshops that you find inspiring, keep up with reading in your professional field, and utilize supervision. • Focus on an area of specialty to deepen your knowledge. • Validate what you already know, give training or papers at conferences.	• Be organized in your private and professional lives. • Set goals. • Follow through on "to-do lists." • Be aware of times your Impulsive/ Undisciplined Child modes are triggered.	• Set aside time for play with friends, your partner or children, pets. • Take time off to engage in the leisure activities that you enjoy. • Schedule such time if needed to ensure that it happens and be open for whatever play appeals to you. • Get friends together for game nights; go to the zoo or an amusement park.

When Your Schemas and/or Modes Are Triggered

Unresolved maladaptive schemas and modes of the therapist might interfere with the treatment process, causing emotional distress for both client and therapist. Following are some examples of therapeutic pitfalls related to therapist maladaptive schemas and modes.

Avoidant Coping Modes

If the therapist has an Avoidant Coping pattern, it may prevent him or her from being open and direct with the client or addressing "hot topics" as they arise during sessions. Avoidance on the part of the therapist can prevent the development of a healthy therapeutic process, leaving the patient openly frustrated and further reinforcing the therapist's avoidant coping. An increase in client frustration might also run the risk of activating maladaptive schemas linked to the Avoidant Coping, such as abandonment, failure, etc., which will add to the emotional distress of both client and therapist.

Overcompensating Modes

A therapist who is overcompensating for various maladaptive schemas might, in contrast to a therapist who uses Avoidant Coping, be too confrontational toward clients. A therapist who is overcompensating for a failure schema might be quick to point out and criticize clients for not being able to follow through on assignments, etc. A therapist overcompensating for a defectiveness schema might make clients feel flawed when revealing private thoughts and behaviors that the therapist dislikes within him- or herself. A therapist overcompensating for emotional deprivation might get angry at a client for bringing up a crisis at the scheduled end of a session for not recognizing the therapist's need for time management (e.g., ending the session to be home in time). A therapist overcompensating for a mistrust/abuse schema might fail to set healthy limits for the client, thereby placing them both in potentially dangerous situations. A therapist with overcompensation issues will run the risk of becoming overly stressed and burned out due to ongoing schema activation during sessions that is not cared for in a healthy manner.

Surrender Coping Modes

A therapist with a Compliant Coping style (i.e., surrendering to his or her schemas) will run the risk of burnout due to not setting needed limits and/or not standing up for his or her own needs. A therapist surrendering to a failure schema might keep putting the blame on him- or herself during sessions if the client is not making progress, instead of placing realistic responsibility on the client for following through on his or her part of the work. A therapist with mistrust/abuse issues might allow clients to criticize and bully him or her instead of setting realistic limits, for example, when working with narcissists. A therapist surrendering to a Self-Sacrifice schema might foster client dependency and eventually have difficulty meeting the client's level or range of needs.

Demanding Critic Modes

Many professionals find some Demanding Critic to be adaptive (e.g., during school, when working to meet deadlines or to complete time-sensitive tasks). However, an ever-present internal Demanding Critic can rob a therapist of job satisfaction, lead to unnecessary frustration with progress or time length of therapy, and undermine therapist confidence and feelings of mastery. This Dysfunctional Critic mode can also cause a therapist to have an imbalance in work versus pleasurable and relationship activities—another path to burnout.

There are several ways for a schema therapist to reduce the risk of maladaptive modes interfering when conducting therapy. The first step is to become aware of how you feel and what mode is triggered. When you are aware of a strong emotional reaction during or after a session, or even when you see a particular client on your schedule, it can be helpful to complete a Self-Monitoring Circle (presented in Module 6). This analysis will give you a lot of information about your experience and help you form a plan to deal with any interfering modes. Of course, we also use our reactions to our clients as important information about how others may respond to them. It is important to sort out what may be a personal reaction we are having from what is likely the general reaction anyone would have to, for example, an Overcompensating Coping mode in our client. Supervision and peer supervision are excellent places to get feedback about and increase awareness of our modes being triggered. This kind of therapist feedback is a central part of ST supervision. Professional and peer supervision are both important sources for therapists to get their needs met (e.g., needs for validation, confidence building, constructive feedback, reinforced competence, acceptance). If you have completed the SP/SR workbook, you may want to go back to the exercises for the mode with which you are struggling and repeat the exercise or reread your self-reflection. If you become aware of more intense triggering in sessions, personal therapy would be an important resource to utilize.

In summary regarding the issue of safeguards, we have tried all the exercises in the workbook with clients (with a wide range of severity of problems), therapists in training, and ourselves. We use these ST interventions, without adverse effects, with patients who have severe BPD who are court-committed to locked psychiatric units, and with people with schizophrenia. We think that the safeguards included here and in Module 1 of the exercises are adequate for people with the amount of Healthy Adult mode to gain acceptance into, or to have completed, an ST training program. Ida likes to say that I am her "guinea pig" for experiential exercises, as she tries new exercises on me first. We have had no negative outcomes from their use, but we have had emotional activation, as that is often their goal. We do not see these exercises as harmful to therapists if the safeguards described in this chapter are used. Becoming a schema therapist requires quite a bit of self-awareness, ability to be open and genuine, and flexibility. Therapists overwhelmed by the exercises of the workbook might want to consider some personal therapy or even another therapy modality. Looking at the positive side of working through the SP/SR program, therapists tell us how valuable the experience has been for their personal growth, solving "stuck points" related to EMS and Maladaptive Coping modes, and how helpful it is in understanding their clients at an emotional level. In our judgment, the benefits vastly outweigh the minor risks.

The Process of Self-Reflection

ST Training

Training and supervision in ST include self-reflection. Therapists monitor their schema and mode activation and have the experience of assessing their own schemas and modes using the YSQ. Most training programs have therapists in training construct case conceptualizations on themselves. Fifteen hours of role-play interactions are included in the individual ST certification training, thereby providing therapists with the opportunity to experience the interventions, gain self-awareness, and increase understanding of clients' experiences. However, as Bennett-Levy et al. (2015) observe, therapists have different levels of natural self-reflective capacity. For this reason, they offer suggestions for Self-Reflective Questions, for preparing for reflection, and for the process of reflection and self-reflective writing. We include a summary of their guidelines in the next sections.

Self-Reflective Questions

Each module finishes with a series of Self-Reflective Questions. They follow a progressively deepening path:

- What was your immediate experience of the exercise? What feeling, bodily sensation, thought, image, and/or memory were you aware of?
- Were you aware of any schema activation or mode triggering?
- What did you learn about yourself—as a person and/or as a therapist? Was the exercise helpful or unhelpful to your process?
- What are the implications of your experience for your understanding of your clients' experiences? For your work with clients? How will you implement this new understanding in your next client therapy sessions?
- How does your experience affect your understanding of ST?

These Self-Reflective Questions move you from personal experience to professional implications. Like CBT SP/SR, ST SP/SR is designed as a targeted, focused training strategy that makes an explicit link between the personal and the professional. This approach to self-practice is consequently different from individual therapy, which focuses primarily on the personal domain.

The modules also have Self-Reflective Questions that inquire about the experience of the specific exercises in each module.

Self-Reflective Guidelines*

Preparing for Self-Reflection

* Schedule a time for reflection rather than waiting until you feel like opening your notebook.

* Be prepared to experience strong emotion—uncomfortable, distressing, exciting, or joyful feelings. There is no correct way to feel; whatever you feel is correct for you.

* Be prepared for times of ambivalence about continuing the work. Do not give up abruptly. Consider which Coping or Critic Mode may be interfering with doing the work. Change takes time and is difficult—that is what we tell our clients.

* Be aware of naturally occurring breaks such as vacations and have a plan for resuming the work.

* Plan where you will keep your notebook to ensure privacy and confidentiality. Some people prefer a physical notebook, whereas others use password-protected electronic files.

The Process of Self-Reflection

* Find a quiet spot where you can be undisturbed for the length of time you plan to use (approximately 30–45 minutes).

* Breathe, focus on your body, get comfortable.

* Reflect on any thought, feeling, or sensation that you have.

* Provide a transition from the self-practice exercise into self-reflection. This transition could involve some focused breathing, connection with your Safe-Place Image, or using the grounding exercises provided in Module 2.

* Find your own way to recall situations and their accompanying emotions, thoughts, bodily sensations, and behaviors. It is usually helpful to close your eyes to focus inwardly. Try to choose a specific situation or memory from the self-practice exercise on which to reflect. You can reconstruct it vividly by recalling the sights, sounds, and smells in as much detail as possible. Some people run a "movie clip" in their minds to

---

*Adapted for ST self-reflection from Bennett-Levy et al. (2015).

recreate the experience. Breathe to the center of your body and check for the physical manifestations of emotion.

- Don't censor your thoughts or question your feelings. Allow enough time for the feelings to develop. If you begin to have a feeling—for example, tears coming to your eyes—do not immediately try to discover what it is about, just let it come. If you move into attempting to analyze the feeling, it may never develop enough for you to discover what it is about. Sometimes feelings do not have content or direct connection to memories. This is particularly true of very early preverbal memories and experiences.

- Be open to being surprised by your feelings. Try to avoid having too many preconceived ideas about what the experience will be like.

- Be aware of Maladaptive Coping modes being triggered—either avoidant ones leading to your detachment, or overcompensating ones leading you to criticize and dismiss the process of reflection.

- Be aware of thoughts that contain the messages or rules of your Dysfunctional Critic mode—for example, that this process is "stupid" or that you are "doing it wrong," or that you are coming up with only inane or superficial reflections. Send the Critic mode out of the room.

- Be gentle and compassionate with yourself. Therapists are human beings; we all have our flaws and strengths. We will experience the same kind of mode triggering our clients do. We cannot be other than human, and our humanness is part of what helps our clients heal.

- Your reflections do not have to be confined to the period you assign to them. You will probably have thoughts throughout the week, and it is helpful to record them in your notebook also.

- There are Self-Reflective Questions throughout the modules that are merely suggestions and are not meant to limit you. You may come up with other cues that aid your reflective process—use them.

- Link the personal and the professional in your reflections. The research by Bennett-Levy et al. (2015) suggests that people who gain the most benefit use SP/SR to reflect on both their personal-self and their therapist-self, going back and forth between the two aspects of themselves.

Self-Reflective Writing

- Write in the first person (i.e., use "I" statements).

- Writing is a core component of the reflective process because writing engages thinking. It can stimulate thoughts in a different way than thinking alone.

- Write for yourself without concern of someone reading it. You will share your reflections only as you choose or not at all. The more honest and open you are, the more you will gain from the experience.

The Three Therapist Examples: Julia, Penny, and Ian

We use examples from the experiences of three "fictional" therapists throughout the modules. These three therapists are combinations of the many therapists we have worked with in SP/SR groups, personal therapy, and ST supervision. Identifying information has been removed or changed to minimize the likelihood of someone thinking we are describing him or her. However, as the examples illustrate common experiences for therapists, their stories may seem familiar. We also use some our own experiences in the examples given for Julia, Penny, and Ian.

We deliberately chose therapists at different points in their careers. Julia is a relatively new therapist in the middle of ST training. Penny is a certified ST supervisor-trainer with more than 20 years of practice. Ian has worked as a therapist for 5 years and has taken one weekend course in ST. He is thinking about whether he will pursue ST certification. All three identify a problem that lent itself to the work of the SP/SR program. In these introductions, we deliberately avoid using ST model language, so that the process of moving from a client's description of his or her problems to an ST conceptualization can be illustrated in the assessment exercises of the modules.

Julia

I am a 28-year-old psychotherapist working two part-time jobs, one in a clinic and the other in private practice. I have an MA in psychology and am licensed in my country as a psychotherapist. I have completed the training component of an ST program and am in weekly supervision. The problems I am aware of are a lack of self-confidence as a therapist and a lot of concern over whether new friends or even new clients will like me. I have difficulty setting limits with my clients and find that sometimes I am not very present in sessions. I often run over the session time. I also have difficulty setting limits when clients are in Bully–Attack mode. After such sessions, I feel distressed and self-critical; I call myself "stupid" and "useless" and end up bingeing on chocolate and sweets to feel better. I feel better briefly, but then I criticize myself again for gaining weight and being fat and disgusting. I have had concerns about being "good enough" since I was a child. These concerns are affecting my relationship with my girlfriend; I do a lot to try to please her, and then I am unhappy and withdraw if she is not as attentive and complimentary as I am. I'm afraid I'm damaging our relationship.

Potential problems I have tentatively identified for my SP/SR work:

1. Detaching in therapy sessions and not being able to set limits
2. Being very self-critical when I am less than perfect or make mistakes
3. Bingeing on sweets to calm unpleasant feelings

Penny

I am a 50-year-old senior clinical psychologist with a PhD. I am married with two adult children. I have been a trainer and supervisor in ST for many years. I am an advocate for SP/SR for my supervisees and continue to apply ST strategies to my own process. I know that I have very high standards for my students, my family, and myself. When I don't meet, them I get very self-critical. I think of extreme criticisms like "You stupid idiot" or "You are useless." I drive myself to work very long hours and try to make things perfect. I also drive my students and demand a lot, often micromanaging their work. I do the same at times with my adult children. I don't want to be so demanding. I am concerned that I may even be demanding with my clients. I am first-generation Japanese, and I think that cultural issues may be involved in my drive and perfectionism. I decided to participate in the SP/SR program now to intensify my work on these issues because they affect my personal and professional lives.

Problems I have identified for my SP/SR work:

1. Pushing myself or supervisees too hard
2. Micromanaging my supervisees
3. Spending so much time trying to perfect my work that I have no time for my family.
4. Being a demanding parent with my clients when they are not working to my standard

Ian

I am a 35-year-old male psychotherapist. I have a master's degree in social work and am licensed as a psychotherapist. I was trained in gestalt therapy and CBT. I recently began training in ST. In the last 6 months, I started a new job and got married, which has increased my overall anxiety considerably. Lately I find that I am very touchy when I am given any negative feedback, or a different way of doing things is suggested to me. My automatic thought is "He/she is saying I'm inadequate, stupid." I often respond with a defensive reaction that is too big for the present situation. On a few occasions, I have even called my wife a "controlling bitch," hurting her feelings, and pushing her away. I notice that some of my colleagues seem to avoid me, and in the training group I am often picked last as a partner.

Problems I have identified for my SP/SR work:

1. I am very sensitive to any negative feedback and get overly defensive and angry when I feel criticized. This reaction pattern happens with supervisors and my wife.
2. When I am very angry with my wife, I call her inappropriate negative names.
3. I am not able to ask my wife directly for the validation and support I need.

The identified problems Julie, Penny, and Ian chose for their SP/SR work will appear throughout the workbook. We can follow their progress in using SP/SR and see how it increases their awareness of feelings, needs, modes, schemas, and choices and provides opportunities for change and healing.

CHAPTER 4

Guidance for Facilitators

In this chapter we share our observations and suggestions from 20 years of facilitating various versions of SP/SR groups. We know of no published studies to evaluate ST SP/SR, although it is extensively practiced. There is extensive research evaluating CBT SP/SR groups (Bennett-Levy et al., 2015, summarized in subsequent sections of this chapter). We can make extrapolations from the CBT findings, but the effects of ST SP/SR groups need empirical validation. We also summarize the findings of the CBT research in terms of the "influencing factors" that have been identified, which we think can be applied to ST SP/SR groups.

Our Own Experience from Participating in Self-Practice Groups

The first experience for both of us in a self-practice group was the one in which we met 32 years ago. We were both practicing psychotherapists engaged in personal therapy with the same psychotherapist, who was also the group leader. The SP group used bio-energetics and gestalt techniques. It was composed of eight therapists and met 1 day a month over a number of years. We both found that this group was helpful in terms of personal growth, awareness of our own triggers in the group setting, increased comfort with our experiential interventions, and increased understanding of client experiences in a group.

We routinely participate in some of the exercises in the SP/SR groups we lead. After 10 years of regularly leading these groups, we still find that we always learn something more about ourselves or clients' experiences.

> ## Example
>
> In an exercise designed to fight the Critic mode, participants shared one of their messages and the childhood experience related to it, followed by sitting in the center of the group circle and hearing from others the messages they deserved to hear. Ida chose the message "You aren't as pretty as your sisters." This perception dated back to her premature birth and having very little hair for her first few years. Her full-term younger sister had beautiful long locks, which her mother was always brushing and curling while commenting on her beauty. The group gave lovely messages to Ida about her worth, value, and beauty. She had not realized until that experience just how much this childhood experience had hurt her and how much the feelings came back at times when she was in the Vulnerable Child mode. She also understood better the intensity of her reaction when looking at baby pictures with Joan, who had thick, shoulder-length, curly masses of hair at the age of 1. She realized that although she laughed when Joan teased her about it, she actually felt hurt. Sharing her feelings led to an apology for the unintended hurt and the end of the teasing.

Experiences like the one in this example and our assessment that we both continue to benefit from participating in ST SP/SR are some of the reasons that we recommend the program with confidence even for experienced schema therapists.

Our Experience Leading Therapist Self-Practice Groups

Based upon our positive experience participating in SP/SR, we set up groups for practicing therapists and for clinical psychologists and psychiatrists as part of their training in group therapy. These groups were originally more broadly experiential, then moved to the ST model 12 years ago. The reports of participants in these groups suggest that SP/SR is an effective tool both for training and for personal self-awareness and growth.

Participating in a ST SP/SR group of at least 1 day is a requirement of the ISST for certification as a group schema therapist. We regularly lead these groups as part of our training programs in individual and group ST. From our contact with James Bennett-Levy and the *Experiencing CBT from the Inside Out* workbook, we added a written self-reflection component. Having to write responses to Self-Reflective Questions gives participants the opportunity to integrate their thoughts and feelings before sharing them. Responding to questions stimulates aspects of self-reflection that therapists may not have considered. For example, the question of how the experience of an intervention adds to their understanding of the model and how the experience affects their understanding of their clients may influence the work they do. This was the kind of awareness that was usually the focus in our SP/SR groups, but it was productive to have these important questions considered by all participants before general discussion. Self-reflection also provides a mechanism for further considering aspects of the experience that therapists may not want to share in discussion, but which could benefit from more thought shortly after the experience. We experimented with a number of different formats for discussion of self-practice experience: the group as a whole, smaller subgroups with subsequent whole-group discussion, and one group member having the responsibility to summarize his or her group's reflections and self-reflection alone without additional discussion. We found that discussion in smaller groups allowed participants to be stimulated by each others' reflections and provided enough time for them to give their comments and then benefit from the later wider discussion with the group as a whole. From our observation, the optimal size for the small group appears to be eight, the size also generally recommended for therapy groups (Yalom & Leszcz, 2005).

Formats for ST SP/SR

1-Day ST SP/SR

The focus here is, of necessity, limited. The group can decide which mode or modes to focus on in self-practice work, based upon the individual needs of those present, or the format could generally follow that of ST client groups. In the latter case, the process would focus on (1) establishing connection and safety; (2) an exercise facilitating awareness of one's default Coping mode; (3) an exercise to diminish the control of the Critic mode; (4) an experiential exercise to address the needs of the Vulnerable Child mode; followed by (5) a short experiential Happy Child exercise; and ending with (6) an exercise to strengthen access to the Healthy Adult mode.

A Sample 1-Day Format for ST SP/SR

Exercises

1. The Safe-Place Image exercise (Module 1).
2. The Safety Bubble exercise, adapted to include the whole group for connection (Module 1).
3. The Problem Analysis exercise to choose a problem on which to focus and identify the roles of the maladaptive modes (Module 7).
4. The Smothering the Critic exercise (Module 17).
5. The Good Parent Script for the Vulnerable Child (Module 16).
6. A Trip to the Toy Store imagery exercise (Module 19).
7. Walking through the Modes exercise to access the Healthy Adult mode (Module 20).

All exercises can be found in the workbook modules listed in parentheses.

Self-Reflective Questions

Each exercise is followed by Self-Reflective Questions and group discussion of the experience.

1. What sensations, thoughts, and feelings were you aware of?
2. Were any schemas activated or modes triggered?
3. What self-awareness did you gain?

4. What did you learn from your experience about what your clients' experiences might be?

5. What did you learn from the experience that you will apply in your work with clients?

2- or 3-Day Weekend Group

In this format, the agendas described above could be extended with added time for self-reflection and discussion and the addition of more than one exercise for each of the mode groups.

12 to 20 Group Sessions

This version could follow the format of this workbook or another strategic plan for the sessions based upon the overall goals of ST. To our knowledge, this format has not been tried, but should be as productive as the CBT SP/SR training programs described by Bennett-Levy et al. (2015). This program should be evaluated in terms of participants' experience: their confidence in doing ST, their increased understanding of the ST model and clients' experiences of the interventions, and their own personal results. This change could be measured with the SMI, with the instruction to participants to base their answers on a specific time period, and possibly with the YSQ. Since the SMI has recorded changes in clients who participated in a 3-month group ST program (Farrell & Shaw, 2016), we would expect positive change in therapists who complete an SP/SR program.

Other SP/SR Formats

For many years Romanova and Kasyanik (2014) have facilitated week-long group programs with clients and therapists that begin at birth, go through childhood and the development of schemas and modes, examine adulthood and the maintenance of schemas, and extends into the future, based on changes participants report from the corrective emotional experiences they have had in the group process. There have been no studies to evaluate this format, but the evaluations by participants is very positive. They report new understanding of their current mode-related problems and a sense of freedom from old patterns.

The Role of the Group Leader

The role of the group leader in ST is always that of a "Good Parent" practicing limited reparenting. Being genuinely present and sharing one's own experiences and emotional reactions as they apply to the needs of the group are all part of ST limited reparenting. This also means taking responsibility, to a varying degree, for the safety and cohesiveness of the group (depending upon the group's needs), and directing the work of the group. When the group is primarily in the child mode, the therapist leader is, in essence, the parent of a young child, giving directions, providing containment and guidance, managing conflicts actively and directly, and meeting attachment needs. When the group is in adolescent modes, the leader will step back and allow more autonomy. When in healthy modes, the leader becomes a facilitator with a more supportive and less directive role. The progression of limited reparenting in a ST group is more fully expounded in Farrell and Shaw (2012).

As suggested for CBT SP/SR (Bennett-Levy et al., 2015), we ensure that participants are clear that it is their decision to engage with SP/SR at whatever level they choose; it is their choice whether or not to publicly report their reflections; and it is up to them to choose the partner with whom they wish to work.

Setting the Stage for an ST SP/SR Program

In looking back on the various versions of SP/SR that we have led, the most successful have been those directly linked to training in ST. In this version participants spend at least 3 days together in didactic and dyadic exercises in which they have the experience of being a client in a ST group with us as the therapists, leading the group as a demonstration of various interventions. The fourth day is the SP/SR day in which the focus of the work shifts to them in the client role. The least successful SP/SR daylong group that we led was one in which most of the eight participants did not know each other at all; the day of the SP/SR program was their first meeting. The organizer of the program had not described the program specifically and had opened it to the general therapy community. The needs of the participants varied considerably: a few wanted to experience ST and others were meeting a licensing continuing education requirement. Even though we ended the day with the nagging feeling that it had not been very successful, the participants' anonymous evaluations were quite positive.

We see this less-than-optimal group experience as an example of a mismatch in expectations: We expected quite a bit of insight from active participation in the group process and exercises; they were not sure what to expect, but apparently what they experienced had met their varied expectations adequately. From these experiences, we learned to be specific in the description and goals for the program and to negotiate directly about these and the structure before beginning. This attention to clarity and specificity regarding the program's content is particularly thoughtful when the program is even a few days in length. Obviously for a 12-day or longer program, having an agreed-upon structure and similar expectations would be critical.

ST Group SP/SR Structure

We conduct an ST SP/SR day in a similar manner to the way we lead client therapy groups. We begin with facilitating the sense of safety and connection that is critical for the vulnerability that ST requires. We assess the needs, goals, and expectations of the individuals in the group and collaboratively plan the work accordingly.

Establishing Safety

- **Therapist commitment to safety:** We state our commitment to keep participants safe in the group process; to set limits as needed; to provide validation of feelings and the need for comfort and support, etc. These behaviors are all consistent with limited reparenting.

- **Public agreement to confidentiality:** All personal content revealed in the group must be kept private. We ask for a show of hands to acknowledge agreement, and we make deliberate eye contact with each member.

- **Choice:** Therapists are encouraged to share as much in the group as they feel comfortable with. Personal content is not necessary; it is enough to identify the modes and/or schemas involved. For pair exercises, participants choose their partners, and for small-group exercises, we let participants assemble the groups, as they wish.

- **Self-care is encouraged:** We strongly encourage participants to top if they feel too much distress or are overwhelmed. We set up a "safety corner" in the group room with pillows and blankets. Participants may go there at any time. The therapist will check in with anyone in the safety corner, acknowledging that the participant is taking care of him- or herself and can rejoin the group whenever he or she wishes. If a long time is spent there or extreme distress is evident (e.g., a flashback of some kind), one of the therapists will offer help or suggest a group effort to help. This extreme response rarely, if ever, happens, but nonetheless it is important to set up the safety conditions to handle it.

Facilitating Connection and Cohesiveness

We begin with group exercises to establish connection among participants and a sense of group cohesiveness. Facilitating connection and cohesiveness is not described in the individual workbook modules, but can be found in Farrell et al. (2014).

- **Circle greeting exercise.**
- **Connecting web:** Yarn is thrown back and forth among the members and the connections are felt by tugging, letting go, etc. The individual connections are identified as representing what is needed in the group, with each participant offering what he or she needs: for example, trust, acceptance, respect, etc. The experience is discussed.

- **Group transitional object:** The therapists give a glass bead on a piece of cord as a symbol of membership in the group. The beads are different in some way and the same in another, which provides an opportunity to discuss the issue of similarities and differences in the group and for the leaders to declare that all are accepted. The participants tie the cords around each others' wrists, which is another experience of contact or connections.

Setting an Agenda

- Group SP/SR programs utilize personal goal setting. The mode model provides a common focus while allowing for individual goals and experiences within each mode exercise.

- We take requests for work on particular modes or schemas and particular interventions, so that the content of the day matches the needs and interests of the participants.

- We set the agenda actively and collaboratively.

Expectation of Benefit

- We share our self-practice experience and highlights from the evaluations of previous groups.

- We summarize the research findings for ST client groups.

- In client groups, we tell members in early sessions that "ST will most likely be the hardest therapy you will ever do, but we can tell you from research findings that if you engage fully, it will also have the biggest benefit—not just on symptoms, but also on the quality of your life." This statement also can be made in the SP/SR group.

- We describe the rationale and potential benefits from the point of view of ST. A "hard sell" is not needed, as therapists interested in ST usually have some idea of how the person of the therapist is involved, so the potential for increased self-awareness appeals to them. Often participants have done some personal therapy or experienced some sessions in their ST supervision.

- We summarize the research findings for CBT SP/SR groups presented by Bennett-Levy et al. (2015) in Chapter 4 of *Experiencing CBT from the Inside-Out: A Self-Practice/Self-Reflection Workbook for Therapists*. Participants gain insight into themselves as "a person" and "as a therapist"; they acquire more confidence in practicing CBT interventions, a better understanding of CBT, and more empathy for and understanding of their clients' experiences. We expect the same benefits from ST SP/SR.

Potential Benefits of the Group Version of ST SP/SR

- Participants can be stimulated by each others' comments to reflect more on their own experiences and their implications for therapy.

- Universality occurs (a common therapeutic factor in groups [Yalom & Leszcz, 2005]). Participants see that others have similar emotional reactions to the exercises.

- A cohesive, effectively working group can increase engagement and deepen the SP/ SR experience by offering additional perspectives and stimulating greater depth of reflection. Engagement is related to positive outcome (Bennett-Levy et al., 2015).

- Participants can benefit from the general therapeutic factors of groups: universality, belonging, acceptance, vicarious learning and information, and re-family effects. Just as limited reparenting provides corrective emotional experiences of Good Parents meeting a child's needs, in a group, clients experience corrective emotional experiences from having a surrogate healthy family that includes the roles of siblings, grandparents, aunts, uncles, and so forth. We refer to this experience as "re-family effects."

- Groups can provide accountability, which increases the completion of assignments and facilitates active involvement.

Potential Problems with the Group Version of SP/SR

Bennett-Levy et al. (2015) identified the following potential problems in the group version:

- Doing programs with workplace colleagues can inhibit engagement.
- Participants may fear of exposure to other participants.
- Participants may fear losing control of their emotions and the high distress that may occur in sharing their reflections with others.

Summary

Combining our experience leading ST SP/SR groups and the empirical findings of Bennett-Levy et al. (2015) for CBT SP/SR, we suggest the following general guidelines for conducting SP/SR groups:

- *Address safety concerns* and create a safe environment. Identify any fears regarding exposure and find ways to address these concerns. Gain public agreement to confidentiality.
- Confirm that all participants have a *Safe-Place Image* and in longer-term groups, a *safeguard strategy.*
- *Distinguish content* (personal information) *and the process* of the exercises. Suggest mode language.
- Make clear that *reflections can be private or public.* Participants can share as much or as little as they choose.
- Facilitate *active collaboration* around the program agenda.

- Ask participants to *identify a challenging personal problem* of moderate to high emotional intensity, which they are motivated to change.
- Address questions about your *role as facilitator*. In ST SP/SR, this is the role of limited reparenting.

Participant Responses to the Group Format of Schema Therapy SP/SR

- "It was useful to have the space to think with others about the impact of the self-practice and self-reflection. It felt like a safe space to do this because there were connections with others, but also the anonymity of not working together on a daily basis."
- "I felt that the small group self-reflections were most useful, as it was good to be able to use others' thinking and understanding of the modes applied to real issues.
- "It was an interesting learning experience for me about the schemas triggered and my feelings and behavior in a group."
- "It's impossible to deeply understand if you don't try it how beautiful it is to have nine people that are behind you, to protect you and to take care of you. I emotionally realized why group ST is so powerful. It gives people a 'new family,' the family they deserve and that they need."
- "The support that you feel in the middle of that circle of people makes you feel safe and able to face the most frightful challenges of your life. I think it would be very useful to introduce into the training more self-therapy to understand even more deeply the amazing effects of group schema therapy."

Responses to the Group Connection and Safety Exercises

- "The circle introduction exercise was a powerful bonding exercise, and promoted the safety of the group. I was surprised at how much more connection I felt and how much it increased my willingness to share my self-reflections."
- "From my experience in the connection exercises, I realized at a felt level how very important it is to have a safe connection as the first goal and a necessary condition for therapy."
- "I learned a lot from my experiences in the group; in the beginning how difficult it can be to tell my own story and later on how it feels to be connected to other group members."
- "I was struck by people's openness and honesty in the self-reflection. It felt like a supportive and nonjudgmental atmosphere."

Group ST SP/SR for a Team of Colleagues

- "I was curious to see how self-therapy would work in a group, especially because we were going to this with colleagues with whom I work. I found that these sessions helped to create a very safe environment."

- "The experience helped the team members to have open communication with each other and to be compassionate and not overly critical when we are working together. I think the clients can feel this sense of safety that we feel with each other. Our openness helps when they are having doubts about staying in therapy or struggling. I think it helps if they can see how we model having a connection between us as therapists because many of them have had so few positive experiences of connection."

Introduction to the Workbook Modules

Each of the 20 SP/SR modules has the following four sections and some have a fifth section: Assignment. The sections can be identified by their titles.

1. **Notes:** This section contains notes to psychotherapists about how this module fits into ST theory, concepts, and interventions.
2. **Example:** Here we give an example of how one of the three therapists we are following through the workbook completed the exercise.
3. **Exercise:** This is the self-practice part of the module. It may contain more than one exercise, which you may want to complete in more than one session.
4. **Self-Reflective Questions:** These questions ask you about your experience of the exercises and how it affects your understanding of ST, your understanding of your clients' experiences, as well as how it will affect your future work with clients.
5. **Assignment:** Some modules have assignments to complete before moving on to the next module. It is important to complete the assignment, just as we tell our clients.

In the workbook we have included examples of the core exercises we use for you to try. You may or may not use all of them with your clients, but you will have had the experience of them and in the future be better able to make the choice that best matches your client. From our use of these exercises in facilitator-led groups, we think that they can generally be completed within 60–90 minutes. This is also the typical length of client group ST sessions. If you find an exercise is taking you longer than that, or you have decided to devote only 60 minutes at a time to the workbook, we suggest that you do only one exercise from the longer modules. In this case, it is important that you complete the Self-Reflective Questions for any exercise just after you complete it.

PART I

Connection and Safety

Setting the Stage
for Schema Therapy Self-Practice

As the title states, the first two modules of the workbook provide exercises and tools to establish the safety and connection needed to do ST SP/SR. Module 1 describes the construction of a personal Safe-Place Image to use to reduce any distress experienced. It also provides instructions for a fantasy-type image: the Safety Bubble. To assist you in accessing your Healthy Adult skills when needed, some Physical Grounding exercises are described. The use of a Google group for connection is discussed. Module 2 contains the assessments used in ST to provide a baseline. These are the World Health Organization Quality of Life measure and selected questions from the YSQ and the SMT, which will allow you to identify your schemas and modes.

MODULE 1

Connection and Safety

When I started working as a schema therapist, I decided I wanted to do my self-therapy in the ST model. I wanted to know firsthand what it's like to do imagery and change chairs and all the techniques we use. The SP/SR work was tremendously helpful to me. I still find that I learn something more about myself when I attend these SP/SR days.

—SP/SR participant

I liked the time that we spent on self-reflection and self-care. It's good to have the importance of this for therapists recognized and discussed. Often, in my experience, self-care is only given lip service without any practical application.

—SP/SR participant

Module 1 sets the stage for the work you will do in ST SP/SR by addressing the foundational issues of connection and safety. As discussed in Chapter 2, the initial phase of treatment in ST focuses on connection and safety. In this module, we describe our efforts to provide you with a connection to us, we guide you in developing a Safe-Place Image, and we provide an opportunity for you to experience the use of a Safety Bubble.

Notes. We approach ST SP/SR work with therapists in the same way we do with our clients: We "set the stage" by establishing connection and safety. It can be difficult to feel connected with the authors of a book. To increase connection, we use first-person pronouns and give some examples from our own experiences (Farrell & Shaw, 2012; Farrell et al., 2014). Readers of our earlier books gave us feedback that this disclosure allowed them to feel some connection to us on a personal level. One reader wrote, "Excuse my familiarity, but I feel like I already know you from reading your book as you share some of your own experiences." Strategic self-disclosure is part of the therapist style of limited reparenting. We do not want to be removed, sterile authority figures, but rather transparent human beings with emotions. Connection is a critical element of ST. Without it, a central intervention of ST—limited reparenting—is not possible. As schema therapists, you must establish connection with your client and safety for him or her. Empathic Confrontation, one of the main interventions of limited reparenting, is not possible without connection. Empathic Confrontation brings to the client's attention the fact that his or her behavior, when in a Maladaptive Coping mode, needs correction because it is not getting the person's need met (and often creates additional problems such as others avoiding dealing with the person, seeing him or her as difficult people). For a client to believe that the intention of empathic confrontation is to be helpful and not critical, some connection (e.g., trust, knowing) must have been established.

SP/SR Google Group

For this SP/SR workbook, we have set up a Google group that we will monitor and respond to questions and comments. We hope that the ability to contact us in this way will be another source of connection and support for you as you take the "leap of faith" of participating in an ST SP/SR program. Connection is part of the foundation of safety. You will also be able to post self-reflections there and hopefully view those of others. A commitment to confidentiality is requested, but we suggest that your posts preserve your privacy by leaving out identifying information.

Creating Safety

Safety is another essential element for doing ST. One way safety is established in ST is through participants' visualization of personal Safe-Place Images. Another part of feel safe is having access to your Healthy Adult mode. Just as we do with our clients, you must have these two safety measures in place before starting the workbook. These tools will be part of your Personal Safety Plan.

EXERCISE. Constructing My Safe-Place Image

In ST developing a Safe-Place Image is an important part of the first stage of treatment. It will be used in work with the Vulnerable Child mode and as a replacement for your default Coping mode. For clients, this can be a difficult assignment as they may not have the memory of a safe place readily available. We give them many suggestions and share one of our own Safe-Place Images. Examples we give include a place in their home such as a bedroom, a place in a trusted relative's home, at school with a protective teacher, a friend's house, and a place in nature. Therapists sometimes need to be creative in assisting with this step. One of our clients with BPD came up with the feeling of the wind against her body when riding her bicycle; another recalled mountain climbing when she reached the top and was alone and felt safe. Joan shares her Safe-Place Image of her grandmother's attic, sitting on a cedar chest surrounded by books and toys. The Safe-Place Image can also be imaginary for those who find no current or historical place.

Clients can choose an imaginary place—outer space, a huge protective tree with a hidden house inside, etc., or they can use the Safety Bubble described in the next exercise.

Instructions: Find a quiet place to sit comfortably where you will not be disturbed. Let an image come to mind that represents a Safe Place to you. Don't push it; just be open to whatever safe image occurs. It can be like a movie scene in your mind's eye, a memory, or recall of a picture. It can be something from your life, from your imagination, or from a book or movie. You can bring anything that is safe and comforting into your image. Make it your own. Don't worry if you have some difficulty at first getting a strong image. It will come. People have different ways of developing an image—some use a picture or photo as a prompt. If you have difficulty imagining a safe place, find a picture that represents it or draw it.

1. What do you **see?**

2. Can you see yourself?

3. How old are you?

4. What else do you see?

5. What **sounds** do you hear?

6. Is there a **smell or scent** in the image?

7. How do you **feel** in this place?

8. How does your **body feel?**

9. Is anyone else there? Remember, only safe people are allowed. Anyone or anything unsafe should be ejected from the bubble now.

Self-talk for the Safe-Place Image includes statements such as "I am safe," "I control this space and no harm comes to me here," "I feel calm," etc. Add your own words:

Name your Safe Place so that you can bring it to mind quickly and easily—for example, "Grandma's house," "the treehouse at home," "Mrs. Smith's classroom," etc.

Although soothing imagery is used in other approaches to psychotherapy, Young (Young, 1990; Young et al., 2003) introduced this specific use of the Safe-Place Image.

EXERCISE. The Safety Bubble

In this exercise, you construct the image of a large bubble of safety surrounding you. We use this exercise when people have difficulty constructing a Safe-Place Image, but it can be useful as an image for therapists to stay present in ST sessions in which their Vulnerable Child is triggered or when a client's intense negative emotion feels triggering. Joan uses the image of a protective cocoon wrapped around her for the same purpose. She developed it in our first BPD ST group, fondly referred to as the "group from Hell"—no reflection on the group members, we were just developing our model for group ST at the time.

Instructions: Imagine a bubble large enough for you to fit inside. Imagine it in any color you like and as beautiful as you want to make it. It is a magic bubble because you can walk in and out of it without breaking it. You can take anything into the bubble that will be soothing to you and help you feel strong and safe. You may let other people in, or you may choose to be by yourself. One thing you may not take into the bubble is anything harmful to you or unhealthy.

After you are able to imagine your bubble and have gone into it with whatever you want, imagine the bubble floating away to wherever you want it to go. You may want to close your eyes and maybe even listen to peaceful music as you float away in your safe bubble. No unhealthy critic voices can get through the magic bubble. You may stay in your bubble for as long as you want to or need to. After you come out of your bubble, relax for a few minutes before you do anything else.

You can also put overwhelming feelings or thoughts into the bubble and let it float away until you feel less overwhelmed. You can then take the feelings or thoughts out, one at a time, to address each and your underlying need.

Notes. Having reliable access to the Healthy Adult mode is another safety measure in ST. This mode is described in Chapter 2. The kind of distress people sometimes experience when doing imagery rescripting or emotion-focused work related to childhood experiences is conceptualized in ST as the experience of being in the Vulnerable Child mode. As previously described, it is in this mode that we feel the fear, sadness, loneliness, and helplessness that was our experience in the related trigger situation as a child. What a person needs when in this mode is connection with his or her Healthy Adult mode, particularly the "good-parent" part of that mode. Physical Grounding exercises are one way to connect with your Healthy Adult mode.

EXERCISE. Physical Grounding

This exercise increases your awareness of the physical sensations of your adult body.

Instructions: Slow down and take a few deep breaths. Now stand with your feet about 12 inches apart, and your knees bent slightly. Put your arms out in front of you, palms down. Slowly raise your arms straight up over your head. Hold this position, then tuck your chin to your chest keeping your head down, and with arms still elevated, slowly bend over until your hands are almost touching the floor. Now, keeping your arms hanging down and your head still tucked in, slowly rise to your full height, keeping your knees slightly bent and rolling up your spine one vertebra at a time. This should be done slowly and gently, not forcing anything, rather, allowing gravity to act on your back as you uncurl. Repeat this exercise twice more, focusing on your breathing, letting go of any body tension, and clearing your mind of intruding thoughts. This exercise is likely to help you feel more grounded—with your feet "planted firmly on the ground"—and feeling more connected with your adult body.

Notes. Using a "Transitional Object" to Strengthen Your Safety Images. The idea of a transitional object originally came from Donald Winnicott in 1953 and is a main construct in attachment theory. A transitional object is any inanimate object that becomes connected with the soothing and safety experienced with one's early caretakers. Common examples of transitional objects for children are a soft blanket and a stuffed animal. ST makes use of transitional objects for the adult client's Vulnerable Child mode as one of the corrective emotional experiences provided by limited reparenting. We use transitional objects frequently, particularly for clients with BPD, but also in ST training. This use was influenced by an experience we had with a client whose Defectiveness/Shame schema was so strong that she felt her presence contaminated others and that she saw a monster when she looked into the mirror. Joan worked with this client individually as well as in our inpatient group ST program. It was very difficult to budge the core beliefs related to her Defectiveness/Shame schema. In a session in which Joan was searching for any experience of feeling "not a monster," the client recalled an experience in Ida's group of making an "identity bracelet." Group members gave each other colorful beads to represent the positive qualities they saw in each other. This client reported that when she was being given these beads and heard how group members saw her, she felt that she had some worth. She was wearing the bracelet, so Joan asked her to put her hand over the beads and revisit that experience. She was able to do so and for the rest of the session felt less defective. This allowed her to do some related imagery rescripting work for her Vulnerable Child. An example of the use of transitional objects in ordinary life is the memento we cherish from an important person in our lives or that reminds us of an important event.

We have been a little surprised in our training groups at how therapists bring back the beads and fleece squares that we give them from one training session or SP/SR day to the next even a year later. It supports the idea that all of us have a Vulnerable Child mode, which, when triggered for whatever reason, needs soothing and safety from the Good Parent part of our Healthy Adult mode. We explore this Good Parent further in the modules on the Vulnerable Child mode (Modules 14, 15, and 18).

✍ EXERCISE. Choosing a Transitional Object

Instructions: We suggest that you choose some object that connects with your Safe-Place Image. Suggestions are a bead on a piece of cord to wear as a bracelet or on your keychain or in your pocket; a small piece of soft cloth like fleece; a shawl or scarf, etc. Use it to augment evoking your Safe Place. Try it for yourself and be open to the result. **Describe it here along with its meaning to you.**

```
```

Summary

You can include your Safe-Place Image, the Safety Bubble, Physical Grounding exercises, and a transitional object to access your Healthy Adult mode in the overall Safety Plan you developed in Chapter 3. As described there, it is important to have this personal safeguard plan in case you become unexpectedly distressed as you use the workbook.

📝 ASSIGNMENT

Practice the safety exercises (Safe-Place Image, Safety Bubble, Physical Grounding, Transitional Object) throughout the week. Write about your experiences here.

```
```

It requires practice for your Safe-Place Image to get stronger and more useful as a healthy coping substitute for the Maladaptive Coping mode. Record your practice on the form below and the situation, mode, and result when you chose to use the Safe-Place Imagery.

SAFE-PLACE IMAGE PRACTICE

Day	Situation	Mode	Result of using the Safe-Place Image

Self-Reflective Questions

Now that you have completed the self-practice safety exercises, it is time to reflect on your experience.

What emotions, physical sensations, or thoughts were you aware of while you were doing the exercises? Was your experience of the imagery exercises different in comparison to the physical grounding exercise? If so, how do you understand the difference?

_____

_____

_____

_____

_____

_____

_____

_____

_____

_____

_____

_____

What did you like or find effective in the exercises? Was there anything you did not like or think did not work well for you?

_____

_____

_____

_____

_____

_____

_____

_____

_____

_____

_____

_____

Were there any surprises or changes by the end of the module?

_____

_____

_____

_____

_____

_____

_____

_____

_____

_____

_____

Is there anything you want to reflect on further during the week?

_____

_____

_____

_____

_____

_____

_____

_____

_____

_____

_____

_____

Has your experience of safety exercises "from the inside" affected the way you might use these exercises with your clients? If this is the case, how will you do things differently?

_____

_____

_____

_____

_____

_____

_____

_____

_____

_____

_____

_____

_____

_____

Establishing Your Baseline

I found it very helpful to look specifically at a problem of my own and how the various modes are involved. It really clarified what I need to work on, and I plan to use it with my clients. I think it will help them pull the various ST concepts together and see how they really impact their lives.

—SP/SR participant

In this module, you will complete baseline assessments of your current quality of life and your experience of EMS and schema modes. These measures provide you with a baseline to use to track change as you move through the SP/SR workbook.

The World Health Organization Quality of Life Questionnaire

The World Health Organization Quality of Life questionnaire (WHOQOL-BREF) is one of the measures used in much of the ST outcome research (Wetzelaer et al., 2014). The 24-item version (WHOQOL-BREF) is a self-report instrument for assessing quality of life that ST research uses (WHOQOL Group, 1998); it focuses on the domains of physical health, psychological health, social relationships, environment, positive feelings, negative feelings, and self-esteem. This measure reflects one of the primary goals of ST: improved quality of life. Completing this questionnaire provides you with a personal baseline and gives you an assessment experience that is similar to what is asked of your clients before beginning psychotherapy. Repeat the measure at Module 13 when you are reviewing your progress and making decisions about further work and at the completion of the SP/SR Program.

If you are interested in, or concerned about, your levels of depression or anxiety, you may want to complete the Beck Depression Inventory (BDI) or the Beck Anxiety Inventory (BAI) at the beginning of using the workbook. These inventories could be repeated at the review points of Module 7 and 13 and at the completion of the workbook.

✍ **EXERCISE.** My WHOQOL-BREF

The WHOQOL-BREF questionnaire is available at *www.who.int/substance_abuse/research_tools/en/english_whoqol.pdf*. Scoring instructions are available in the manual found at *www.who.int/iris/bitstream/10665/63529/1/WHOQOL-BREF.PDF*. Norms to interpret your scores can be found in Hawthorne, Herrman, and Murphy (2006).

After completing the questionnaire, enter your scores on the following chart.

MY SCORES ON THE WHOQOL-BREF

Date/Time	Domain	Score	Severity
Initial ratings	Physical		
	Psychological		
	Social Relationships		
	Environment		
At Module 13	Physical		
	Psychological		
	Social Relationships		
	Environment		
Final rating	Physical		
	Psychological		
	Social Relationships		
	Environment		

Caveat: *If you have rated yourself as being in the severe range, we would advise you to consider consulting your supervisor, a knowledgeable friend, your physician, or your therapist if you are currently in psychotherapy. You also need to consider whether this is the right time for you to engage in SP/SR. As you use the workbook, it is important to be as gentle with yourself as you are with your clients and to practice good self-care. Psychotherapists frequently have high scores on the Self-Sacrifice schema and take good care of everyone at the expense of their own well-being.*

The Young Schema Questionnaire

EMS, as they are defined in ST, are assessed using the YSQ. We have taken questions from the YSQ—Short Form (Young, 2017), a self-report instrument containing 75 items that are scored on a 6-point Likert scale. This instrument is used to measure the presence or absence of 18 core maladaptive schemas at the time of assessment. The YSQ is highly sensitive in predicting the presence or absence of psychopathology (Rijkeboer, van den Berghe, & van den Bout, 2005). For SP/SR purposes, we are assessing 10 of the full 18 EMS using two representative YSQ questions for each. We chose the 10 EMS that we find most often in our schema therapist SP/SR groups and in our supervision of psychotherapists. With clients, we recommend administering the full YSQ. For a full EMS self-assessment, you can complete the YSQ-L3 Long Form or YSQ-S3 Short Form. These questionnaires are available from the website *www.schematherapy.com*. If you are or have been involved in an ST training program, you may have already completed the YSQ. If so, still complete the questions here, then compare the result to your previous YSQ results. Note any changes. Since schemas are thought to be similar to personality traits, they may still be present even after psychotherapy but activated less or with less severity.

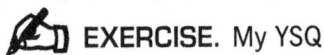 EXERCISE. My YSQ

Instructions: Listed in the form beginning below are statements that a person might use to describe him- or herself. Please read each statement and decide how well it describes you. When you are not sure, base your answer on **what you emotionally feel,** not on what you think to be true. Choose the highest rating from 1 to 6 that describes you and write the number in the space after the schema description. You are asked to respond twice—once to how the schema fits your personal life and second to how it affects your professional life.

MY YSQ (SELECTED ITEMS)

UNTRUE OF ME			TRUE OF ME		
Completely 1	Mostly 2	Slightly 3	Slightly 4	Mostly 5	Completely 6

P1 = Personal Life; P2 = Professional Life	P1	P2
ABANDONMENT/INSTABILITY		
When I feel someone I care for pulling away from me, I get desperate.		
Sometimes I am so worried about people leaving me that I drive them away.		

EMOTIONAL DEPRIVATION		
For the most part, I have not had someone who really listens to me, understands me, or is tuned into my true needs and feelings.		
Most of the time, I haven't had someone to nurture me, share him/herself with me, or care deeply about everything that happens to me.		
DEFECTIVENESS/SHAME		
I am too unacceptable in very basic ways to reveal myself to other people.		
I'm unworthy of the love, attention, and respect of others.		
SOCIAL ISOLATION/ALIENATION		
I'm fundamentally different from other people.		
I always feel on the outside of groups.		
FAILURE		
I'm not as talented as most people are at their work.		
I don't feel confident about my ability to solve everyday problems that come up.		
ENTITLEMENT		
I feel that what I have to offer is of greater value than the contributions of others.		
I hate to be constrained or kept from doing what I want.		
SELF-SACRIFICE		
I'm the one who usually ends up taking care of the people I'm close to.		
Other people see me as doing too much for others and not enough for myself.		
APPROVAL/RECOGNITION SEEKING		
Unless I get a lot of attention from others, I feel less important.		
It is important to me to be liked by almost everyone I know.		
EMOTIONAL INHIBITION		
I am too self-conscious to show positive feelings to others (e.g., affection, showing I care).		
I find it hard to be warm and spontaneous		
UNRELENTING STANDARDS		
I try to do my best; I can't settle for "good enough."		
I can't let myself off the hook easily or make excuses for my mistakes.		

The Schema Mode Inventory

The SMI (Young et al., 2007) is a self-report instrument that consists of 143 items on 16 schema modes that are scored on a 6-point Likert scale. It measures the extent to which dysfunctional as well as functional schema modes are present at the time of assessment. For SP/SR purposes, we have selected two representative items for each of 12 modes. We also suggest that you score items based upon the last 2 weeks, rather than just the current moment, as this will give as a more representative assessment of your mode activity. In general, schema modes are more sensitive to change than schemas because the modes measure your current state. They have been found to change after ST (Farrell & Shaw, 2010), and you may well experience some change after completing the SP/SR program. In Module 5 we examine the meaning of your scores and how they are related to the problem you identified to work on and the plan of that work.

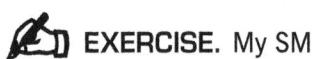 EXERCISE. My SMI

Instructions: Listed in the form beginning below are statements that people might use to describe themselves. Please rate each item based on how often you have believed or felt each statement **in general** over the last 2 weeks, using the numeric frequency scale.

MY SMI (SELECTED ITEMS)

FREQUENCY: In general	
1 = Never or Almost Never	4 = Frequently
2 = Rarely	5 = Most of the time
3 = Occasionally	6 = All of the time

P1 = Personal Life; P2 = Professional Life	P1	P2
VULNERABLE CHILD MODE		
I feel fundamentally inadequate, flawed, or defective.		
I feel lonely.		
ANGRY CHILD MODE		
I have a lot of anger built up inside of me that I need to let out.		
It makes me angry when someone tells me how I should feel or behave.		
IMPULSIVE CHILD MODE		
I say what I feel, or do things impulsively, without thinking of the consequences.		
I have trouble controlling my impulses.		

UNDISCIPLINED CHILD MODE		
I don't discipline myself to complete routine or boring tasks.		
I get bored easily and lose interest in things.		
COMPLIANT SURRENDERER		
I try very hard to please other people in order to avoid conflict, confrontation, or rejection.		
I let other people get their own way instead of expressing my own needs.		
DETACHED PROTECTOR		
I feel indifferent about most things.		
I feel detached (no contact with myself, my emotions, or other people).		
DETACHED SELF-SOOTHER		
I like doing something exciting or soothing to avoid my feelings (e.g., working, gambling, eating, shopping, sexual activities, watching TV).		
In order to be bothered less by my annoying thoughts or feelings, I make sure that I'm always busy.		
SELF-AGGRANDIZER		
I'm demanding of other people.		
I have to be the best in whatever I do.		
BULLY–ATTACK		
I demand respect by not letting other people push me around.		
I belittle others.		
DEMANDING CRITIC (PARENT)		
I don't let myself relax or have fun until I've finished everything I'm supposed to do.		
My life right now revolves around getting things done and doing them "right."		
PUNITIVE CRITIC (PARENT)		
I deny myself pleasure because I don't deserve it.		
I can't forgive myself.		
HAPPY CHILD MODE		
I feel loved and accepted.		
I feel spontaneous and playful.		
HEALTHY ADULT		
I can solve problems rationally without letting my emotions overwhelm me.		
I have a good sense of who I am and what I need to make myself happy.		

Interpretation Grid: Divide the score for each mode by 2 and enter it in the column "Your Score." Next circle the number in each row that your score is equal to or less than.

Mode Name	Your Score	Very Low	Average	Moderate	High	Very High	Severe
The Innate Child Modes							
Vulnerable Child		1	1.47	1.98	3.36	4.47	6
Angry Child		1	1.81	2.29	3.09	4.03	6
Impulsive Child		1	2.15	2.68	3.05	4.12	6
Undisciplined Child		1	2.27	2.87	3.47 (2.95)	3.89	6
Maladaptive Coping Modes							
Compliant Surrenderer		1	2.51	3.07	3.63 (3.32)	4.27	6
Detached Protector		1	1.59	2.11	2.95	3.89	6
Detached Self-Soother		1	1.93	2.58	3.32	4.30	6
Self-Aggrandizer		1	2.31	2.90	3.49 (2.63)	4.08	6
Bully–Attack		1	1.72	2.23	2.74 (2.21)	3.25	6
Dysfunctional Critic Modes							
Demanding Critic		1	3.06	3.66	4.26 (3.71)	4.86	6
Punitive Critic		1	1.47	1.86	2.75	3.72	6

Healthy Modes (high scores are positive)					
	Your Score	Very Low	Low	Average	High
Healthy Adult		2.77	3.60	4.60	5.16
Happy Child		2.11	2.88	4.52	5.06

Notes. You should note any scores in the "high" or "very high" range and include them in the Self-Conceptualization of Module 5. If you have no or few scores in that range, consider those in the "moderate" range for your conceptualization. This system uses the findings of Lobbestael et al. (2010), who analyzed SMI results for a sample of 863 participants, including 319 nonpatient controls without psychopathology, 136 patients with DSM-IV Axis I disorders, and 236 patients with DSM-IV Axis II disorders.

The cutoff scores were determined in the following manner:

- Very Low and Severe equal the maximum score possible
- Average = the mean for the non-patient population
- Moderate = one standard deviation (*SD*) over the mean of the non-patient population
- High = the mean for the Axis II patient sample
- Very High = one *SD* over the Axis II sample

For the Healthy modes, high scores are positive, thus the scores were determined as below.

- Very Low = one *SD* below the mean of the Axis II sample
- Low = the mean of the Axis II sample
- Average = the mean of the non-patient sample
- High = one *SD* above the mean of the non-patient sample

You will use your YSQ and SMI scores in Module 5, in which you develop your ST Self-Conceptualization.

Identifying Your Challenging Problem for the SP/SR Program

The next step is identifying a challenging problem on which to work for SP/SR. This problem can come from your professional work or "therapist self" or from your personal life or "personal self"—or the problem you choose may overlap both areas of your life.

Notes. Psychotherapists are not superhuman people. We all struggle with some effects from our schemas and modes. In addition, the practice of ST may entail more vulnerability in the therapist due to its requirement for a strong personal presence—being there as your genuine self as well as a psychotherapist. Situations in which others are evaluating your competence may cause discomfort and activate early maladaptive schemas. Supervision, group supervision, peer supervision, presenting cases in team meetings, presentations at conferences, giving trainings, meeting a new client—are all common situations in a psychotherapist's life that can be triggering. Look over the examples of common therapist problems in the next gray box and then read the "challenging problems" our three illustrative therapists (Julia, Penny, and Ian) identified that follow. As noted, we use their examples throughout the workbook to illustrate the SP/SR exercises.

There are many potential situations that occur in administering psychotherapy to which we may react personally: clients' canceling sessions, dropping out prematurely, not improving; and clients with diagnoses such as borderline or narcissistic personality disorder. Our clients' impaired and troubled ways of responding interpersonally will occur in their relationships with us as well. Some of these interactions will parallel those with which we struggle in our personal lives and activate our schemas. Clients' use of overcompensating defenses can be hurtful or trigger our own overcompensating modes.

Examples of Professional Problems: Your "Therapist Self"

- You find yourself worrying or ruminating about your work.
- You feel upset before, during, or after therapy sessions, lectures, or supervision.
- You feel like an "impostor" in your professional role—the fear that someone will expose you and see you for the "incompetent" therapist you fear you are.
- You have concerns about personal adequacy—for example, "Am I warm and genuine?," "Am I believable in the 'good-parent' role for my client?," "Am I able to comfort my client?," "Can I meet my client's needs within professional boundaries?," "Am I able to set needed limits in a 'good-parent' manner?"
- You are sensitive to clients' negative personal reactions to you.
- You feel uncomfortable using exercises that elicit strong negative emotion in the client or working with strong emotions, whether angry or sad, ashamed, etc.
- You are self-conscious regarding your application of unfamiliar experiential exercises. For example, you struggle between staying in your chair doing cognitive work or getting up and initiating a mode dialogue using multiple chairs.
- You may find that working with clients who have certain diagnoses or are from certain age groups makes you feel anxious.
- You may see clients who are struggling with some of your own past or present issues, such as death or divorce.

Examples of Personal Problems: Your "Personal Self"

- Being too much of a follower in a relationship.
- Social anxiety.
- Difficulty dealing with interpersonal conflict effectively.
- Fears of abandonment in important relationships.
- Boredom.
- Loneliness.
- You may experience states of anxiety, sadness, and anger and have accompanying physical sensations or symptoms related to one, two, or all three of them.

 EXAMPLES: The Challenging Problems Chosen by Julia, Penny, and Ian

Julia: <u>My identified problem</u> is to be able to set limits and boundaries with clients and deal more effectively with critical or angry behavior.

Penny: <u>*My identified problem*</u> *is having unrealistic demands for myself and others and being perfectionistic. I have no time for fun or leisure activities, and I cannot enjoy successes because I think that I could "always be better."*

Ian: <u>*My identified problem*</u> *is my behavior when I am anxious or angry at home and with supervisors at work. My behavior seems to be out of proportion to the immediate situation. It is alienating my wife and affecting my evaluations at work.*

EXERCISE. My Problem to Work On

Instructions. Choose a challenging problem that occurs in your professional or personal life or one that has some effect on both. In preparation for this exercise, find a quiet space for yourself where you will not be disturbed for the time you need.

1. Allow any emotions or thoughts about yourself as a therapist that worry or upset you to come to mind.
2. If you are choosing a personal problem to work on, allow those feelings and thoughts to come to mind.
3. Bring to mind the emotions, images, and thoughts about yourself as a therapist that may worry or upset you—or about yourself as a person, if you have decided to focus your SP/SR on your "personal self." (See Chapter 3 for guidelines around selecting a "therapist issue" or "personal issue.")
4. We all have our own triggers. Can you identify situations in which you think your emotional reaction is, or was, particularly strong or out of character? We all can run up against unhealthy or ineffective patterns of behavior in our client or personal relationships. Like our clients, we may feel "stuck" with automatic responses to triggers that feel out of our control.

MY CHALLENGING PROBLEMS OR SITUATIONS

---

5. Evaluate the situations you have identified. Choose one that causes you a moderate to high level of emotion (e.g., anxiety, frustration, anger, or distress).
6. Finalize your challenging problem and describe it in the following box.

MY PROBLEM TO FOCUS ON FOR THE SP/SR PROGRAM

Self-Reflective Questions

What stood out or was surprising to you in completing Module 2 of the workbook?

_____

_____

_____

_____

_____

_____

_____

_____

_____

_____

_____

_____

What was your immediate emotional reaction to doing the assessment exercises? Were you aware of any thoughts or physical sensations?

_____

_____

_____

_____

_____

_____

_____

_____

_____

_____

_____

_____

_____

After your experience of rating your quality of life, EMS, and schema modes, what are your thoughts about this process for your clients? Has your experience of this assessment "from the inside" changed the way you might do this with your clients? If this is the case, how will you do things differently?

_____

_____

_____

_____

_____

_____

_____

_____

_____

_____

_____

_____

_____

How easy or difficult was it to articulate your problem? Does your experience give you any added insight into your clients' experiences? Will you approach identifying the problem to work on any differently as a result of your experience?

_____

_____

_____

_____

_____

_____

_____

_____

_____

_____

_____

_____

_____

_____

Is there anything else that you noticed that you would like to keep reflecting on during the next week?

_____

_____

_____

_____

_____

_____

_____

_____

_____

_____

_____

_____

_____

_____

Understanding Your
Identified Problem
Using Schema Therapy Concepts

The three modules of Part II focus on understanding the origins of your EMS and schema modes and their relationship to the current life problem on which you have selected to work in the SP/SR workbook. We have several different ways to approach gathering this information—some cognitive and others experiential. In **Module 3** you will explore your experience of core needs being met (or not) in childhood and adolescence and how they are met (or not) today via a questionnaire. In **Module 4** you will respond to a story about a young child's experience of a need not being met. You will identify the messages she took away from this experience and the gaps in emotional learning that occurred. You will also assess some of your related childhood experiences using an imagery exercise. In **Module 5** you will integrate the information and awareness gained in the first four modules into a Schema Self-Conceptualization.

 Notes. As described in Chapter 2, the ST model of etiology asserts that EMS develop when the basic emotional needs of childhood are not met adequately in the early environment. The role of unmet childhood needs in the development of psychological problems is described in Chapter 2. Childhood and adolescent history are important in ST in that problematic behavior in the present is seen as being based upon faulty learning from normal needs not being met, or gaps in emotional learning from a frustrating or even toxic early environment. ST begins with finding the "root" of a problematic response and identifying the underlying unmet need. ST theory asserts that it is the activation of this need in the present via schemas that leads to the problematic behavior of the maladaptive schema modes. Providing this education and awareness allows clients to understand why and how their Maladaptive Coping responses developed, evaluate their current effectiveness, and decide whether they are willing to change. Young has referred to this approach as working from the bottom up, in contrast to the top-down direction of CBT approaches. The ultimate goal is to help clients get their needs met in an adaptive manner.

Understanding the Development of Your Early Maladaptive Schemas

This questionnaire was a real surprise for me. I thought that most of my childhood needs were met, but in going over them specifically with the questionnaire, I remembered some of the times that I had needed reassurance and no one was there. I got a distinct memory of how often I was left with babysitters. I remembered crying and holding on to my mom's skirt and her telling me to be a big girl. I can see this exercise really helping with clients who have a big Detached Protector mode about their childhood.

—SP/SR participant

In Module 3 you will assess how your normal childhood needs were met, or not, and to what degree. In Chapter 2 we described ST's model of the etiology of psychological problems in terms of how core childhood needs were, or were not, met. Consequently, there is a lot of emphasis in ST on identifying these needs. The core needs can be summarized as:

- Secure attachments to others (includes safety, stability, nurturance, and acceptance)
- Autonomy, competence, and sense of identity
- Freedom to express valid needs and emotions
- Spontaneity and play
- Realistic limits and self-control

Notes. Our clients rarely have accurate information about core needs. Some clients gloss over their childhood experiences or idealize their childhoods. Others respond strongly to the very mention of needs. Our group members with BPD were frightened and angry when we first introduced the topic. They said things such as "I hate that word—it was having needs that got me into trouble as a child" or "I'm too needy—that's what I was always told." Some say, "Yeah, I know I had a bad childhood, but what can you do about it now?" We use a simple questionnaire to assess how the five core childhood needs were met, or not, for you in childhood and adolescence and how the adult versions of these needs are met, or not, in your life today. In the assessment phase of ST we consider clients' experiences with each of these needs and help them connect them with their maladaptive schemas. Table 2.2 (p. 12) presents the hypothesized relationships among unmet need, childhood environment, and childhood and adult expressions.

An Assessment of Childhood, Adolescent, and Adult Needs

 EXAMPLE: Assessment of Penny's Needs

> ***Autonomy, competence, and identity development***
>
> *Childhood experience with this need:*
>
> My mother thought there was a "right way" to do everything and that was her way. She told stories proudly of all the advanced tasks that I was able to perform at a younger-than-usual age—for example, ordering my own meal in a restaurant at 2 years old was one of her tall tales. I had to be "perfect" since she had to be perfect, and I was a reflection on her. As a baby or very young child she moved into a separate bedroom from my father, and took me with her, because, she said, I "would not tolerate sleeping in my crib alone." She only moved out and I got my own bed when my brother was born just after my third birthday.
>
> *Adolescent experience with this need:*
>
> I rebelled and wanted to be as unlike my mother as possible. She was very critical of clothing choices, hairstyle, friends, music, etc. I remember when I started parting my long straight hair in the middle, as was the style at the time, and she told me I looked "like a witch." Not being like her still did not give me any validation for my competence or identity. I had my own room, but my mother always kept things of hers in at least one drawer of my dresser that she would have to come in and "check on."
>
> *How I try to meet this need now:*
>
> Boundaries are an issue for me—I can feel definite limits I don't want crossed with my partner and friends. I sometimes overreact to actions that feel like boundary invasions. This behavior can feel intimidating and off-putting to others.

 EXERCISE. My Needs Assessment

Instructions: Look at the following list of core childhood needs. How were these needs met in your childhood? How were they met in adolescence (ages 12–18)? For the needs that still exist, how do you try to meet them today?

1. **Safety and attachment, predictability, and love**

   Childhood experience with this need:

   Adolescent experience with this need:

   How I try to meet this need now:

2. **Autonomy, competence, and identity development**

   Childhood experience with this need:

   Adolescent experience with this need:

   How I try to meet this need now:

3. **Freedom to express my own feelings and needs**

Childhood experience with this need:

Adolescent experience with this need:

How I try to meet this need now:

4. **Freedom to play and be creative**

Childhood experience with this need:

Adolescent experience with this need:

How I try to meet this need now:

5. **Realistic limits and self-control**

Childhood experience with this need:

Adolescent experience with this need:

How I try to meet this need now:

EXERCISE. My Unmet Needs and Related Schemas

1. Locate your unmet needs on Table 2.2 (p. 12) and identify the related proposed schemas. List them here:

   Unmet needs:

   Related schemas:

2. Are any of these schemas ones that you scored high on in Module 2? Which ones?

3. Understanding the relationship between the schemas activated by particular situations and their relationship to unmet needs, past and present, is an important step in gaining the awareness needed for change. We follow up with the information you collected in Module 3 when we develop your Self-Conceptualization in Module 5.

Self-Reflective Questions

What was it like for you to look back at your experience of having needs met, or not, during childhood and adolescence? What feelings, thoughts, and physical sensations did you experience during this exercise? Were any schemas activated or modes triggered?

_____

_____

_____

_____

_____

_____

_____

_____

_____

_____

_____

_____

_____

Did any memories or images come to mind as you worked on the exercise? Record them here:

_____

_____

_____

_____

_____

_____

_____

_____

_____

_____

_____

_____

Were there any surprises?

_____

_____

_____

_____

_____

_____

_____

_____

_____

_____

_____

_____

What have you learned about your client's experience of doing this same work? Has your experience led to you planning any change in the way you obtain and work with this material with clients?

_____

_____

_____

_____

_____

_____

_____

_____

_____

_____

_____

_____

MODULE 4

Stories of Childhood Experience and Assessment Imagery

> The wonderful metaphors (stories) allow you to reach internal parts that need attention. I saw myself in the thunderstorm story. I noticed how my Detached Protector mode works in relation to clients and in my life.
> —SP/SR participant

In Module 4 we explore your experience of having core childhood needs met or not met at the experiential level. In the first exercise, we recount the story of a little girl named Ella experiencing a severe thunderstorm for the first time and the effects of her needs not being met. The second exercise explores your experience of needs not being met in historical imagery and asks you to identify the messages about yourself, other people, or the world that you took away from these experiences.

Notes. We use the stories of childhood experiences in which needs were not met to introduce clients to the process of identifying the faulty and critical messages they took away and the consequent gaps in emotional learning as these form the foundation of early maladaptive schemas and schema modes. Whereas the needs assessment of Module 3 asked you about your experiences related to core childhood needs, asking you to respond to a story adds an experiential component to this assessment. The story approach seems to engage clients more easily in the task of observing the effects of well-intentioned parent behavior on children. Discussing unintended negative effects from parenting helps diffuse the family loyalty issues that sometimes arise. Most clients find a childhood memory of a need not getting met fairly easily. It is also easier for many clients to accept and defend the needs of a character in a story than those of their own. The use of imagery makes the ST theory of the etiology of psychological problems more salient and real.

EXERCISE. The Story of Ella and the Thunderstorm

Instructions: Find a quiet place where you will not be disturbed, read the story, and then answer the questions that.

"A little child 4 years of age woke from the crackling and banging sounds and loud rumbling of a thunderclap that was so loud she felt like it was shaking her bed. Bright flashes of lightning, which left behind scary images on the walls, followed the loud noises. At the next thunderclap she flew from her bed and ran to her parents' room feeling so frightened that all she could do was shake and cry. Her crying turned into a scream at the next sound of thunder. One parent woke and started to yell at her. "Stop crying," the parent said, "it's just a thunderstorm. Stop being such a big baby! Go back to bed before you wake the entire household." Ella went back to her room but couldn't stop crying. She bit down on her blanket so no sound would escape. She tried covering her ears so she wouldn't jump at the thunder, and she closed her eyes to stop seeing the scary arms that were reaching out to grab her from the walls. She bit down harder, kept her eyes closed, and blocked her ears every time the thunder came. After a while she didn't jump any more, even though the thunder was louder, nor did she shake and duck when the creepy arms tried to get her. She just sat there staring off into space."

Consider the following questions and answer them by filling in the chart on page 103.

1. What did Ella feel as she was running to her parents' room?
2. What did she need?
3. What did Ella feel after her parent's response?
4. What message about herself (feelings, needs, worth), the world, and other people would Ella have taken away from this experience?
5. What modes do you think were triggered or began to develop for Ella?
6. What would you expect the effects to be on her adult life if similar experiences occurred repeatedly?

Scene	Feelings	Needs	Messages	Modes	Adult effects?
In Ella's bedroom as she prepares for sleep					
Goes to parents' bedroom					
Ella returns to her bedroom					

✍️ **EXERCISE.** My "Good-Parent" Response to Ella

Instructions: What would a "Good Parent" response to Ella that addressed her needs look like? Write out your suggestions in the following box, as we will refer to it later when we work on developing Good Parent messages and actions for you. Here we just want you to start thinking about how Little Ella's needs could have been met.

📌 *Notes.* Ella's story provides an example of the kind of situations in childhood in which needs were not met and the resulting responses contribute to the development of EMS and Dysfunctional modes. It demonstrates the vulnerability of children and the gaps in emotional learning that can occur in the absence of parental guidance and information. The situation does not need to be one of outright abuse, but rather a time when a child was left on his or her own to deal with intense feelings before he or she had the brain development, information, or resources to do so. To cope with such situations, a version of the fight, flight, or freeze, response will occur—that is, a Maladaptive Coping mode—and thus the problematic development begins. One of the most common child responses in the thunderstorm story is that of the Detached Protector mode. Repeated experiences in which needs are not met strengthen this coping mode.

This exercise also provides a safe example for clients of how negative messages begin, and it helps them move on to identify their own negative messages. The messages that we take away from our childhood and adolescent experiences form our core beliefs about ourselves, other people, and the world—the cognitive aspect of EMS. These messages are not necessarily spoken, but rather inferred from the way we are treated and how our core childhood needs are responded to. These beliefs can be positive and healthy or negative and unhealthy. They may be based upon unrepresentative experiences: those unique to a family (e.g., "in our family no one ever gets less than an A grade on a test"), or held by a particular cultural group (e.g., cultural beliefs about the value of girls), temporary circumstances (e.g., a childhood illness and separation due to hospitalization), or a traumatic experience of abuse. Those early messages may not accurately reflect your current reality, but they do affect your adult experience because they are accepted at an intrinsic level as "truths." They can act as "self-fulfilling prophecies" either by distorting your interpretation of experience or by filtering out experiences that contradict them. The imagery rescripting exercises of Module 19 have the goal of changing those core beliefs that were internalized from experiences of core childhood needs not being met.

Assessing Related Childhood Experiences through Imagery

Now we would like you to go a step further in identifying the childhood experience related to your identified problem by visiting one of your related early experiences in imagery. **We suggest that you not choose a memory of physical or sexual abuse at this point**, but rather one in which you needed a "Good Parent" and no one was there for you.

 EXAMPLE: Ian's Assessment of His Related Childhood Experiences through Imagery

As I read the Ella example, I remembered several times when I was confused and scared and went to my father for comfort and guidance, but he said that I was "being a baby" and that he was "too busy to stop and coddle" me because I "should know what to do." I remember a time when I was 6, playing in our front yard with my little brother of 4, and a stranger came into the yard. I felt frightened and ran into the house to get my father. After I told him what had happened and that I was scared, he yelled at me for leaving my little brother all alone with a stranger and told me to get back out there and tell him to come into the house. I said I was too scared because of the strange man, but he said, "Don't be a baby—you're the oldest and you need to protect your brother." The message I took away was that it was wrong to feel scared or to ask for help. I should have all the answers. So today when I don't have the answers, I think I must act like I do and challenge anyone who questions my performance. This message is part of my Defectiveness/Shame and failure schemas. I think that when these schemas are activated, I overcompensate and get defensive or even attacking of the person who questions me. This is a problem with clients at times, as I get defensive when they question me about something, and I get sarcastic and say things like "Oh, so when did you get your psychotherapist license?" I sometimes call my wife names when she questions how I have done something.

 EXERCISE. Assessing My Related Childhood Experiences through Imagery

Instructions: First make a brief connection with your Safe-Place Image. Close your eyes and get an image of yourself as a young child feeling and needing things similar to what Ella felt—the need for safety, comfort, reassurance, protection, information, etc. Stay with the feelings for a minute or two and then come back and answer these questions.

1. What was your little child feeling? What does he or she need?

2. How were your little child's needs and feelings responded to?

3. What message did you take away about yourself? About other people?

4. Which of your EMS is this childhood experience connected with?

5. Which survival coping strategy did you use in childhood to deal with your unmet needs, just as Ella used one to protect herself: fight, flight, or freeze? How is that early coping strategy related to a coping style you use today? (Refer to Chapter 2 for descriptions of the Maladaptive Coping modes.)

6. Are any of the schemas or modes that you identified from your childhood experience involved in your identified problem? If so, how?

Self-Reflective Questions

What was the experience of doing the imagery exercise like for you? Thoughts? Feelings? Physical sensations? If you experienced any emotional distress, how did you deal with it? Were there any surprises?

_____

_____

_____

_____

_____

_____

_____

_____

_____

_____

_____

_____

_____

Did any other memories or images come to mind as you worked on the exercise? If so, record them here:

_____

_____

_____

_____

_____

_____

_____

_____

_____

_____

_____

_____

How was the experience of reading Ella's story different from retrieving your own memory? Was there less interference from schemas or modes in reading Ella's story than from your own story?

_____

_____

_____

_____

_____

_____

_____

_____

_____

_____

_____

_____

From your experience of these different approaches to assessing childhood experiences—questionnaire, story, or imagery—which did you find most useful? Which would you use first with your clients? Would the approach that you select depend upon the client?

_____

_____

_____

_____

_____

_____

_____

_____

_____

_____

_____

_____

_____

_____

What have you learned about your clients' experiences of doing this same work? Has your experience led you to plan any change in the way you obtain information about, and work with, the needs of your clients?

_____

_____

_____

_____

_____

_____

_____

_____

_____

_____

_____

_____

_____

Your Schema Therapy Self-Conceptualization

The Self-Conceptualization was useful in increasing my awareness of mode development and activation. It also provided a good summary of much of the work we had completed in the didactic portion of the training, and relating that to the self. I have been able to think about my own modes using the exercise, and as a result I have also been more confident in working with clients on their conceptualizations.

—SP/SR participant

In learning the model and interventions, it's very useful to connect the curriculum with your own experiences. In practicing schema therapy, it is also essential to know one's own schemas and modes. It helps the capacity to empathize when you have a sense of how a particular mode or schema feels and what thoughts belong to it. If therapists have had the experience of identifying their own modes, they have a better felt sense of what is helpful, and can better help their patients understand their modes.

—SP/SR participant

In general, by about the fourth to sixth session of ST, therapist and client formulate a Self-Conceptualization (also referred to as a "case conceptualization"). This is a collaboratively created document that is expanded and modified over the course of treatment. In time-limited ST an abbreviated version of this conceptualization form may be used. Refer to Chapter 2 (pp. 10–18) for descriptions of the various schemas and modes. This conceptualization brings together the information that you collected from the assessments of Modules 2–4. In Module 2 you assessed your EMS and modes by answering short forms of the YSQ and SMI. Your YSQ results provide the information needed for section 6 in the blank form on page 116. Your SMI scores provide the information you will need to list the modes related to your identified problem in section 9. In Module 3 you answered the "My Needs Assessment" exercise questions, which provide the information you will need for sections 3 and 4 (p. 115). The following section provides Julia's filled-in form.

JULIA'S ST SELF-CONCEPTUALIZATION

1. My identified problem:
My problem is both professional and personal. I feel incompetent as a therapist, despite successes. I am unable to take in positive feedback, and I blame myself if a client struggles or quits therapy prematurely. This insecurity is also present in my personal life. I wonder if I am good enough for my partner, sometimes even for my friends.

2. My related life pattern:
Doubts about being good enough have plagued me from early childhood. They have kept me from taking risks with challenges at work or toward forming possible friendships.

3. Developmental origins of EMS

Core childhood need	How was it met, absent, or excessive in your early environment?
Secure attachment, which includes safety, stability, nurturance, and love	Little nurturance from father, conditional from mother
Autonomy, competence, sense of identity	Nothing I did was good enough for my mother. I would think I did a good job and then Mom would tell me all of the things wrong with it. I felt wrong because I did not see the flaws.
Freedom to express valid needs and emotions	This did not happen much in my family. Our primarily Anglo-Saxon background is related to some stoicism.
Acceptance and praise	I heard more about what I did wrong than right. I felt like a pest to my brother; I was not wanted.
Realistic limits and self-control	Limits were quite strict, and a lot was expected of me.

4. Family members: Significant events and personality style or temperament of core figures relevant to quality of attachment

Mother	She is a physician who expected high achievement, was intolerant of any difficulty with school, and was impatient whenever I needed help.
Father	Physician also, primarily absent, unemotional, demanded quiet and no problems in family when home; frequently told me I was overreacting.
Siblings	My brother is 5 years older, very successful, the "Golden Child," with little emotional expression, though popular socially. He had little involvement with me, and I felt that he considered me a "pest."
Other significant figures (teacher, family member, peers, etc.)	Teachers also expected a lot from me. Peers teased me about being "Teacher's pet" because I tried so hard to be perfect.

5. Relevant temperamental/biological factors:
Sensitive, somewhat introverted

6. Most relevant EMS linked with developmental origins

Schema	Developmental origin
Defectiveness/Shame	*Response to mother's messages and brother not wanting to include me*
Approval Seeking	*Response to not having my need for validation/ acceptance met by either parent or brother*
Emotional deprivation	*Response to father*

7. Core childhood memories or images: List some specific memories or images likely to be relevant for EMS formation or attachment history.

I remember a time in second grade when my mother was helping me with homework and I was slow in getting it. She looked disgusted and just left, going off to her room and closing the door.

I came home with a "B" once and she asked, "What is this? No daughter of mine gets B grades!" She didn't speak to me for the rest of the day. I think I was in sixth grade.

Another memory is about my dad when my first pet, a parakeet, died. Dad said, "Why are you upset? We can just buy another one." He really didn't understand my crying and wanting to have a burial service. I was in second grade. I got the message that my feelings were wrong.

I have many memories of my brother kicking me out of our rec room so he could be there with his friends. He was mean about it, saying, "I don't want my dumb little sister hanging around."

8. Current EMS triggers: What situations or feelings trigger schema-related reactions in you?

- *Running into difficulty with a client in a therapy session when I do not immediately know what to do, particularly in response to angry modes.*
- *Being asked a question in group supervision or presenting my cases.*
- *Being home alone on a weekend and having strong feelings of loneliness, sadness.*

9. My schema modes and behaviors

Avoidant mode and behaviors

I avoid exposure as incompetent by keeping a low profile at work so that I am never asked to take on something challenging. I refer clients with BPD who I think may be difficult for me on to other clinicians, even though my thesis was on treatment for BPD.

I don't initiate doing things with friends to avoid expected rejection.

I detach in therapy sessions when I am uncomfortable.

Mode involved: *Detached Protector*	**My name for it:** *"Airhead"*

Surrender mode and behaviors *I accept that I am not good enough, that I am incompetent, and that eventually others will discover this. I accept that no one wants my company and that I am doomed to be alone.*	
Mode involved: *Surrender to Defectiveness*	**My name for it:** *"Little Dummy"; that is how I felt Mom thought about me, although she never actually called me that.*

Overcompensating mode and behaviors *I work fanatically on case notes, treatment plans, etc., so that they will be perfect and I will not be criticized or exposed as incompetent.*	
Mode involved: *Perfectionistic Overcontroller*	**My name for it:** *"Slave Driver"*

Child modes

Vulnerable Child mode experience: My feelings, thoughts, behaviors *Lonely and anxious*
My name for it: *"Little Julie"*

Angry or Impulsive/Undisciplined Child mode experience: My feelings, thoughts, behaviors *I am not really aware of feeling angry. I think I'm afraid of it.*
My name for it:

Dysfunctional Critic Mode experience: My feelings, thoughts, behaviors *Demanding and Punitive Critic—berates me for all my imperfections, says I am worthless, lazy. incompetent and no one cares about me.*
My name for it: *"The Dictator"*

My Healthy Adult mode's strengths and abilities

- *I know I am intelligent because I completed graduate school.*
- *I am a kind and caring person, empathic with others.*
- *I am responsible; my clients can count on me.*
- *When I am not feeling insecure, I can be very present in therapy sessions.*
- *I am hardworking.*
- *I am unselfish.*
- *I am a loyal friend.*

🖊 **EXERCISE.** My ST Self-Conceptualization

Now it is your turn to begin work on your ST Self-Conceptualization on pages 115–118. Some of you may already have done this in your ST training program. If so, take a look at your original form and update it here, if needed.

MY ST SELF-CONCEPTUALIZATION

Date:

1. My identified problem:

2. My related life pattern:

3. Developmental origins of EMS	
Core childhood need	**How was it met, absent, or excessive in your early environment?**
Secure attachment, which includes safety, stability, nurturance, and love	
Autonomy, competence, sense of identity	
Freedom to express valid needs and emotions	
Acceptance and praise	
Realistic limits and self-control	

4. Family members: Significant events and personality style or temperament of core figures relevant to quality of attachment	
Mother	
Father	
Siblings	
Other significant figures (teacher, family member, peers, etc.)	

5. Relevant temperamental/biological factors:

6. Most relevant EMS linked with developmental origins	
Schema	**Developmental origin**

7. Core childhood memories or images: List some specific memories or images likely to be relevant for EMS formation or attachment history.

8. Current EMS triggers: What situations or feelings trigger schema-related reactions in you?

9. My schema modes and behaviors

For the listed modes, if you have not named them, do so now, as in Julia's example.

Avoidant mode and behaviors	
Mode involved:	**My name for it:**

Surrender mode and behaviors	
Mode involved:	**My name for it:**

Overcompensating mode and behaviors	
Mode involved:	**My name for it:**

Child modes
Vulnerable Child mode experience: My feelings, thoughts, behaviors
My name for it:
Angry or Impulsive/Undisciplined Child mode experience: My feelings, thoughts, behaviors
My name for it:
Dysfunctional Critic Mode experience: My feelings, thoughts, behaviors
My name for it:

My Healthy Adult mode's strengths and abilities
•
•
•
•
•
•
•
•
•
•

My Happy Child mode behaviors
•
•
•
•
•

EXERCISE. A Visual Display of My Modes

In ST, we often use a visual representation of the four categories of an individual's modes as an abbreviated visual summary and a working document that can be updated as change occurs. Clients can get a bit overwhelmed with the multiple-page conceptualization and prefer the one-page visual of the change they have accomplished. Penny's mode map is shown on page 119. A blank form for you to complete with the content of your mode categories is found on page 120.

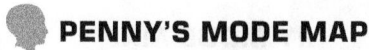 **PENNY'S MODE MAP**

FUNCTIONAL MODES

Moderate healthy adult
Little happy child

MALADAPTIVE COPING MODES

Perfectionistic Overcontroller—
Nothing is good enough, it can always
be improved.

I drive my supervisees so hard
that I have heard they dread
meeting with me.

I spend hours a day
making sure everything is in order.

Detached Protector—
When my VCM is triggered,
I sometimes just withdraw,
stay home and pet my dogs.

DYSFUNCTIONAL CRITIC MODES

Demanding Critic—"Sister Ann"

Work harder, stay up late to go over
those slides one more time—
I drive myself.

I am critical of others' work also,
but don't tell them.

INNATE CHILD MODES

Vulnerable Child—
I just want Mom to love me.

Angry Child—Go away I hate you.
On rare occasions I have a bit
of a temper tantrum
when something is not right.

MY MODE MAP

FUNCTIONAL MODES

MALADAPTIVE COPING MODES

DYSFUNCTIONAL CRITIC MODES

INNATE CHILD MODES

Self-Reflective Questions

What was your overall immediate reaction to doing your Schema Self Conceptualization? Were you aware of any emotions, bodily sensations, or thoughts while you were filling it out? Were there any surprises?

_____

_____

_____

_____

_____

_____

_____

_____

_____

_____

_____

In this module, you have used the mode model to understand your identified problem. What new information have you gained? What are the main things you would like to remember from the first five modules? Make a list of the points that you want to recall in your personal life and in seeing your next clients.

_____

_____

_____

_____

_____

_____

_____

_____

_____

_____

_____

_____

Which exercises in Modules 1–5 were most helpful in adding to your understanding of yourself? Which were least helpful? What are the implications of your experience for your work with clients?

_____

_____

_____

_____

_____

_____

_____

_____

_____

_____

_____

_____

Describe your experience of self-reflection so far. Have you had any difficulties with the workbook? Is there anything you need to do to make things easier for yourself?

_____

_____

_____

_____

_____

_____

_____

_____

_____

_____

_____

_____

_____

_____

PART III

Planning Change
Self-Monitoring, Problem Analysis, and Goals

The modules of Part III are designed to assess the current operation of modes, which are involved with your identified problem, and to set goals for each mode. Awareness of when and how your schemas are activated and your mode states are triggered today is a necessary, though not sufficient, step of behavior change. The self-monitoring techniques of **Module 6** provide you with the means of detecting early warning signs of modes being triggered so that you can make a conscious choice about how to respond, instead of defaulting automatically to a maladaptive mode behavior, which does not get your needs met. You will also construct a pie chart, which provides a visual representation of your overall current mode experience. In **Module 7** you will analyze your problem in terms of the mode activity you have identified and set goals for each mode involved.

The Operation of Modes in Your Current Life

I really liked the monitoring form. I was surprised at how much I learned about my schema activation and mode triggering just from completing one circle. I think I can be more convincing now in motivating my clients to use this tool.

—SP/SR participant

In Module 6 we move from the past and the origins of EMS and dysfunctional modes to the present in terms of their effects on your life now. In the first exercise, we ask you to collect information about your experience of activated schemas and triggered modes using an abbreviated mode diary: the Self-Monitoring Circle. You will continue monitoring activations related to your identified problem for the rest of the SP/SR program. In the second exercise, we ask you to approximate the proportion of time in your daily life that you spend in each mode category. This monitoring provides important information for the Problem Analysis and Change Plan of Module 7.

You may decide to complete each exercise in a separate time slot.

Notes: Schema and Mode Awareness. Education about childhood needs and the impact of those needs going unmet is the first level of awareness work in ST. The next level of awareness is the ability to be aware when schemas are activated and when they trigger dysfunctional modes. In self-practice it is important to be aware of the presence of a Child mode and to take advantage of that opportunity to meet the need with the good-parent skills of your Healthy Adult mode.

As your awareness increases, mode behavior will not be as automatic and you will have a window of opportunity to choose a more effective behavior. Through collecting and recording information about your emotional experience—the schemas and modes that are triggered; the situation, physical sensations, need, feelings, and thoughts—you will be able, over time, to gain improved self-understanding and control dysfunctional mode behavior. Mode awareness in ST is a necessary, though not sufficient, component of change work. This component is further described in Chapter 2. In later modules we add the other two essential components: mode management, which focuses on behavioral pattern-breaking work, and experiential mode work, which focuses on the emotional level.

Clues That a Schema Has Been Activated or a Mode Triggered

1. **Your emotional reaction feels "bigger"** to you than the immediate situation you are in, in the present. You experience high levels of emotion, although it is not a survival situation.
   - "I hate _____."
   - You are passive–aggressive and talk about a problem with one person with others to influence them negatively about that person.
   - You recognize that some of your feelings are familiar—for example, you recognize their childhood origin.
   - Other people you respect give feedback or respond nonverbally as if your reaction is "too big" for the situation you are in.

2. **You feel misunderstood.**
   - This could mean that you are reacting in an idiosyncratic way to a situation because of your personal history and the schemas that were activated by the situation, thought, or feeling you had in the present. The same situation might be neutral for someone else because he or she did not experience what you did. The fact that your emotional reaction is different than others' reactions does not make you wrong. You may want to change your reaction, however, if it does not get the response you want or it leads to not getting your need met.

3. **You realize that a cognitive distortion is involved**—for example:
   - All-or-none thinking: "You *always* do _____"; "You *never* encourage me."
   - Catastrophizing: "This is terrible"; "I cannot stand this for a minute."
   - Negative forecasting: "Because this happened, I will never succeed"; "They will never understand."
   - Cognitive distortions are one of the processes that maintain EMS.

Keep these clues in mind as you begin your Self-Monitoring Circle exercise.

ST Self-Monitoring: The Circle

The first self-monitor form that we use is in the shape of a circle. One of Ian's Self-Monitoring Circles is shown on page 129.

IAN'S SELF-MONITORING CIRCLE

SITUATION–SCHEMA

Fight with wife
Failure

SCHEMA MODE

VCM, ACM,
Bully-attack,
Detached protector

PHYSICAL AWARENESS

Jaw tight, flushed,
shoulders tight

UNDERLYING NEED

To be appreciated, respected
Feelings validated

WANTS

To do things my way
without question

CHOICES TO MEET NEED

Stop talking, leave room
Say hurtful things
Tell her how I feel and what I need
Apologize for yelling at her

THOUGHTS

I don't deserve this,
how date she?

ACTION TAKEN

I told her I felt disrespected
I needed to be listened to
I apologized for yelling

FACTS

She was trying to be
helpful, I am very
sensitive to even
perceived criticism

FEELINGS

Hurt, angry

RESULT: Was your need met?

Really good result, she told me how she felt,
we came up with a code word to use when this happens
in the future. Yes.

Notes. You may wonder why chose a circle, rather than the usual linear forms used in other therapy approaches. We have found that clients, particularly those with BPD, will complete circles with much less resistance than the usual linear monitoring forms. We speculate that the visual representation of movement around a circle from one aspect of their experience to another is somehow more understandable to them and more engaging. This speculation was reinforced when Joan decided to put boxes on the circle so that their writing could be more neatly contained. The patient group objected strongly. We have learned over the years to yield to preferences of this type. Using a circle also distinguishes this monitoring from the many other types our clients have typically experienced, reducing complaints that "I've done this before and it didn't help." We have clients begin by just recording their situation and their awareness of any accompanying feelings, thoughts, and actions and only later add in the other categories, such as mode, facts, etc. Using the Self-Monitoring Circle in therapy sessions allows a focus on the critical elements of experience rather than getting bogged down with lots of content. We want to know how clients felt and what they needed, not the color of dress their mother wore and the weather when she yelled at them. It is part of the socialization process in ST—leading clients to focus on the core aspects of their problems in terms of schemas, underlying needs, and dysfunctional modes.

EXERCISE. My Self-Monitoring Circle

Instructions: Complete the blank Self-Monitoring Circle on page 131 for a situation or experience related to your identified problem from the last few weeks.

MY SELF-MONITORING CIRCLE

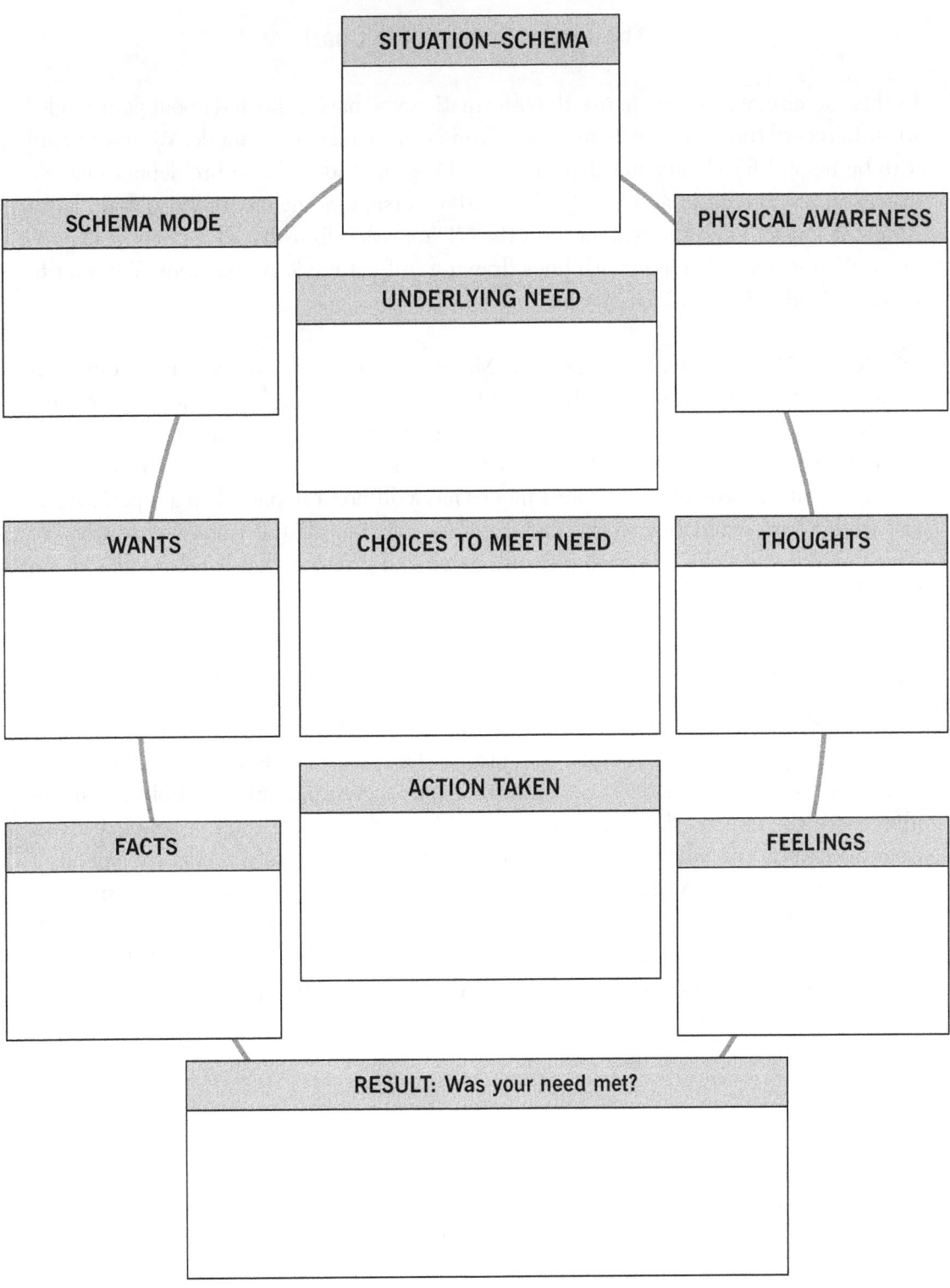

SITUATION–SCHEMA

SCHEMA MODE

PHYSICAL AWARENESS

UNDERLYING NEED

WANTS

CHOICES TO MEET NEED

THOUGHTS

ACTION TAKEN

FACTS

FEELINGS

RESULT: Was your need met?

The Mode–Schema Pie Chart

In this exercise, we ask you to use the information you have collected about your modes so far to record the approximate amount of time you spend in each mode. We have found it to be helpful for clients and therapists working on mode-related problems to have a visual representation in addition to the written version. Somehow the visual aid has a different impact and is consistent with the ST approach to using all aspects of experience. We use a simple circle with lines drawn to reflect mode proportions. We refer to this as a Mode–Schema Pie Chart.

 Notes. We have clients complete the Mode–Schema Pie Chart early in therapy—as soon as they are able to monitor their modes and schemas—and then again at review points throughout their treatment. When working with clients who have many schemas, we simplify by focusing on modes and not listing schemas on the chart. We find that having a visual representation of one's modes has a different impact than a typed listing, as noted. ST is "foundation work," and it will feel at times like it is moving slowly. We have found that it helps to have a measure of general progress that is recorded and can be pulled out as evidence of positive change.

EXAMPLE: Julia's Mode–Schema Pie Chart

Julia's Mode–Schema Pie Chart is shown on page 133. It represents the proportion of time in her typical day-to-day functioning that she spends in the modes related to her identified problem. Julia's chart indicates that she is spending quite a bit of time struggling with the effects of the Demanding Critic mode, feeling quite a bit of distress. As indicated by the Vulnerable Child mode and the Angry Child mode, she spends a significant amount in Maladaptive Coping modes—about the same amount spent in Healthy Adult and Happy Child modes. It is not surprising that Julie experiences a high degree of engagement in the SP/SR program. We will have to monitor her distress level to ensure that her symptoms don't require some individual therapy intervention.

JULIA'S MODE–SCHEMA CHART #1

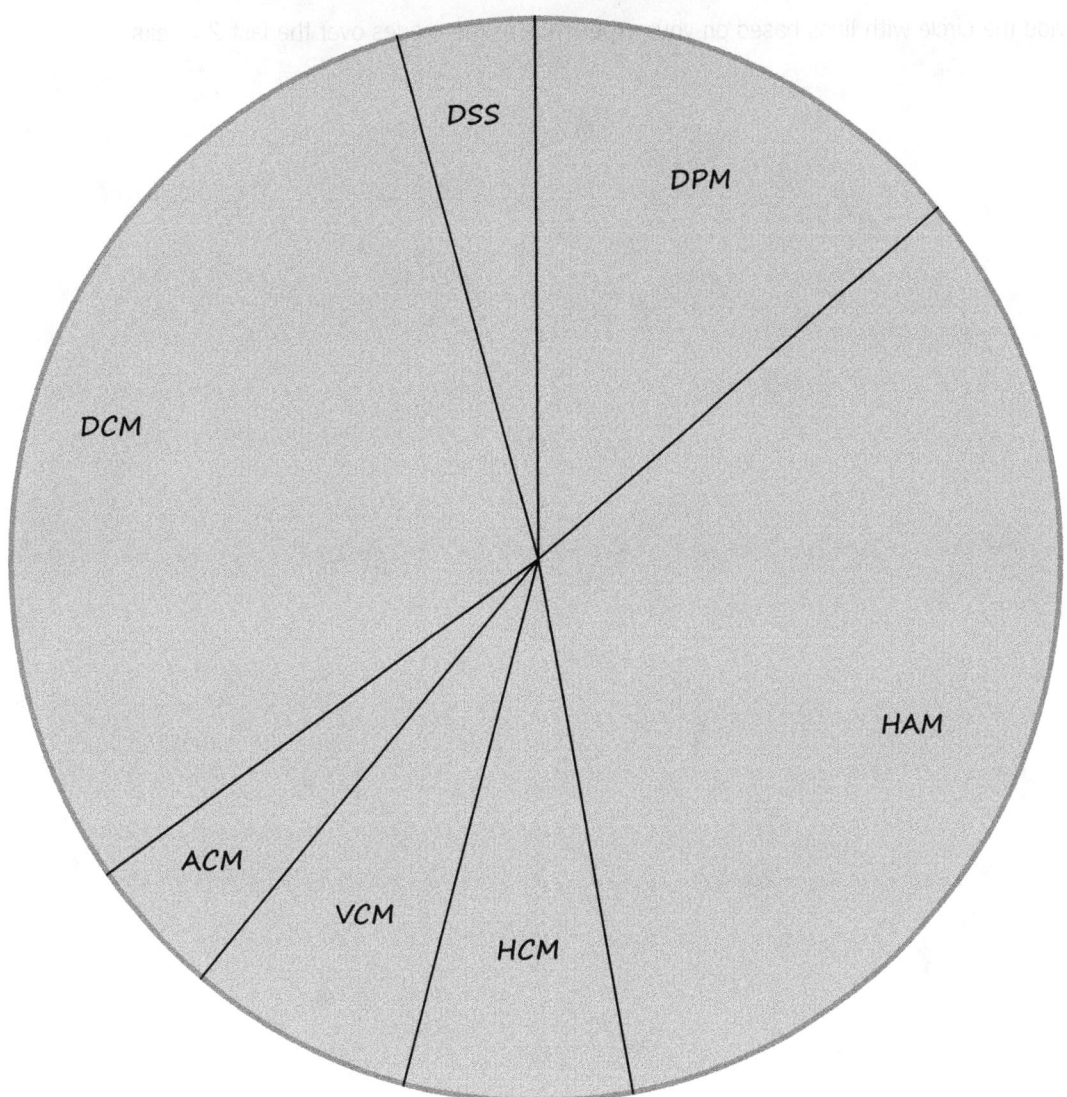

Mode labels key: VCM, Vulnerable Child; ACM, Angry Child; DPM, Detached Protector; DSS, Detached Self-Soother; DCM, Demanding Critic; HAM, Healthy Adult; HCM, Happy Child.

✍ EXERCISE. My Mode–Schema Pie Chart

Instructions: Construct your Mode–Schema Pie Chart using the form on page 134. Modes are the immediate, current state we are in and thus can change from moment to moment. For this purpose, we are asking what your mode states have been like proportionately over the last few weeks, as related to your identified problem. Using lines, indicate on the circle the proportion of your time spent in particular modes. You do not have to use all the modes, just the ones that you experience. Then in the box list the EMS that you determine may be triggers for the modes.

MY MODE–SCHEMA CHART #1

Date: _____

Divide the circle with lines based on your experience of the modes over the last 2 weeks.

Mode labels key: VCM, Vulnerable Child; ACM, Angry Child; I/UCM, Impulsive/Undisciplined Child; DCM, Demanding Critic; PCM, Punitive Critic; AVM, Avoidant Coping Modes; DPM, Detached Protector; DSS, Detached Self-Soother; OCM, Overcompensating Coping Modes; POC, Perfectionistic Overcontroller; BAM, Bully–Attack; SAM, Self-Aggrandizer; AAP, Attention/Approval Seeking; CSM, Compliant Surrender Modes; PCM, Punitive Critic; DECM, Demanding Critic; HAM, Healthy Adult; HCM, Happy Child.

In Module 13 you will be asked to repeat this exercise. We find that it is important for clients to have a tangible representation of their progress through ST, particularly those who have dichotomous thinking and conclude that there is no change unless *everything* has changed. We suspect that it is also helpful for therapists to have this visual display.

ASSIGNMENT

For the next 2 weeks try to do at least one circle per day. When you become aware of a "clue" that a dysfunctional mode is operating, take time to consider whether a schema has been activated and a mode triggered. "Do a Circle" on the experience. Another alternative is to do a Circle on a time when you have any intense emotional experience (one that you would rate as anywhere from 6 to 10 on a 10-point scale). If the emotional experience is one related to your identified problem, do the Circle monitor on that experience. Otherwise, any intense emotional experience will do. The act of filling out the Circle should lead you to identifying the mode and need.

Self-Reflective Questions

What was your experience of the Self-Monitoring Circle exercise? Was it helpful or not? Were you aware of any schema activation or mode triggering while doing the exercise?

_____

_____

_____

_____

_____

_____

_____

_____

_____

_____

_____

_____

_____

Were you able to identify times where you responded to difficult emotions with a coping mode? If so, how did it feel to have this awareness and what did you do in response to it?

_____

_____

_____

_____

_____

_____

_____

_____

_____

_____

_____

_____

Have you noticed any changes in awareness from doing the Self-Monitoring Circle? How can you maintain this increased awareness of the modes triggered and their effects?

_____

_____

_____

_____

_____

_____

_____

_____

_____

_____

_____

_____

_____

What was it like to see your own Mode–Schema Pie Chart? Were there any surprises in your reaction? Did you experience any schema activation or mode triggering?

_____

_____

_____

_____

_____

_____

_____

_____

_____

_____

_____

_____

_____

What are the implications of your experience for your understanding of your clients'
experiences? For your work with clients?

_____

_____

_____

_____

_____

_____

_____

_____

_____

_____

_____

_____

Your Schema Therapy Change Plan

I found the Problem Analysis form helpful to understanding the relationship of modes and the problem I identified to work on in SP/SR. It gave me the "big picture." I am eager to use this tool with my clients now.
                                                                —SP/SR participant

Having the experience of identifying my underlying schemas, their activation, and the triggering of various modes as a client is extremely helpful to being able to understand and connect with my clients around this experience.
                                                                —SP/SR participant

In Module 7 you will use the information you have collected about your schemas and modes related to your identified problem to develop your ST self-practice change plan.

 Notes. When working with clients, it is important to very clearly link schemas and modes with the problem they present to engage them as active collaborators in treatment. If after the conceptualization session, your client still says some version of "Why do we keep talking about these modes?," then you have not adequately explained the links. The exercise on page 141 takes you through the steps of this process of linking and planning change in terms of modes.

ST Problem Analysis

Before moving on to your Problem Analysis, review Julia's example on page 140.

EXAMPLE: Julia's Problem Analysis

Julia's Problem Analysis identifies the schemas and modes that are involved with her identified problem and influence the action she usually takes. Once she identifies the underlying need of her Vulnerable Child mode, she can see that her Maladaptive Coping mode action does not meet it and that her Critic mode increases both the need involved and her distressed feelings.

JULIA'S PROBLEM ANALYSIS

1. My Identified **PROBLEM**	I have difficult staying present in therapy sessions and setting limits, when needed, in my professional life.
2. **SCHEMA**(S) involved	Defectiveness/Shame, Self-Sacrifice
3. **Activating Situations**	New clients, clients in Overcompensating modes
4. What is my underlying **NEED**?	Acceptance, competence, and validation of my needs
5. How is the **VULNERABLE CHILD MODE** involved?	I feel anxious when I need to implement new interventions. I feel like I am doing something wrong when I limit Bully–Attack mode behavior in clients. Sometimes I even feel frightened.
6. Is another **CHILD MODE** involved? How?	Impulsive Child—sometimes if I am anxious, I say too much about myself to get approval.
7. Is a **CRITIC MODE** involved? How?	Yes—it says I should not feel anxious or frightened and that I look like a fool and incompetent—I should be embarrassed.
8. Is a **MALADAPTIVE COPING MODE** involved? How?	I either detach and go into my head or flip into Attention/Approval Seeking
9. What do you usually do and what is the **RESULT**?	If I detach in the session, I miss where the client is at and am not effective in limited reparenting. I feel bad about my skills as a therapist. If I flip to approval seeking I don't set limits but allow the client to go overtime or I don't stop Bully–Attack toward me.
10. Is your underlying **NEED MET**?	No—all my negative evaluations of my competence are reinforced. I think that my client sees this and I feel even sadder and more anxious.

EXERCISE. My Problem Analysis

Instructions: Use the information about schemas and modes that you collected in Module 2, your ST Self-Conceptualization from Module 5, and your Self-Monitoring Circle from Module 6 to complete the Problem Analysis form beginning below.

1. Fill in your **identified problem,** as you now understand it.
2. Answer the **schema(s) involved** question by considering your highest scores on the YSQ items of Module 2 and from your Self-Monitoring Circle of Module 6. Which are the most relevant to the problem you have chosen to work on?
3. List the **activating situations** in which your identified problem occurs.
4. What **need** underlies the problem?
5. **Vulnerable Child mode:** What strong or disproportionate feelings are you aware of, which seem too big for the present situation alone?
6. **Other Child mode:** Do you take any impulsive or undisciplined action that does not consider the potential negative consequences?
7. **Critic mode:** Are you aware of a critical internal voice that tells you in some way that what you feel is wrong or that you are bad or some other negative label? Do you hear that what you are doing is not good enough or that you never do enough?
8. **Maladaptive Coping mode:** List the action you usually take when the schema(s) you identified is activated. Does this action involve one of the coping modes (Avoidance, Overcompensation, Surrender)?
9. **Result:** How does the dysfunctional mode behavior you identified affect your personal and/or professional life?
10. **Need met:** Is the underlying need you identified in question 4 met? If not, how is that need affected?

MY PROBLEM ANALYSIS

1. My Identified **PROBLEM**	
2. **SCHEMA**(S) involved	

3. **Activating Situations**	
4. What is my underlying **NEED**?	
5. How is the **VULNERABLE CHILD MODE** involved?	
6. Is another **CHILD MODE** involved? How?	
7. Is a **CRITIC MODE** involved? How?	
8. Is a **MALADAPTIVE COPING MODE** involved? How?	
9. What do you usually do and what is the **RESULT**?	
10. Is your underlying **NEED MET**?	

Setting Goals by Mode

After you have identified the negative effects of schemas and modes on your current life, it is time to plan for change. In ST, the overall goal is to be able to get your core needs met as an adult in a healthy manner. As discussed in Chapter 2, the ST approach assesses a problem in terms of all three levels or aspects of a person's experience—cognition, emotion, and behavior—and uses interventions that address each level. In the next exercise, we will analyze your identified problem in terms of your underlying need, how each mode is involved, and set initial self-practice goals by mode. This analysis ensures that the client and therapist have a shared definition of the problem—a critical step in working collaboratively.

 EXAMPLE: Julia's Goals by Mode

As you can see in Julia's example below, the goal for the Maladaptive Coping mode is a behavior, the goal for the Critic mode is focused on thoughts, and the goal for the Child modes addresses emotions. This multifaceted approach of ST allows all aspects of a person's experience to be addressed utilizing behavioral pattern-breaking, cognitive, and emotion-focused interventions.

JULIA'S GOALS BY MODE

Vulnerable Child	*To be able to calm "Little Julia" and reassure her that I can protect her.*
Angry/Impulsive Child	*The same as above. If I am not so nervous, I will be less impulsive.*
Dysfunctional Critic Mode	*To be able to stop my Critic voice and access the Good Parent of my Healthy Adult mode.*
Maladaptive Coping Mode	*To notice detachment beginning and be able to stay present, allowing my Good Parent to soothe Little Julia and access my Safe Place.*
CHANGE PLAN: First Steps	
Healthy Adult Mode	1. *Learn to access the Good Parent skills I use with others to soothe Little Julia.* 2. *Stop my Critic and provide more reasonable Healthy Adult perspective. For example, remind myself that these situations are difficult for me, I am a beginner, but I am doing better and am increasing my competence.* 3. *Take some deep breaths to stay present; feel my feet on the ground and the strength and size of my Healthy Adult.*

EXERCISE. My Goals by Mode

List an initial goal for each of your involved modes in the form below. The initial plan that you develop here will continue to evolve and be refined as your awareness and mode management strategies increase through completing the exercises in the remaining modules.

MY GOALS BY MODE

Vulnerable Child	
Angry/Impulsive Child	
Dysfunctional Critic Mode	
Maladaptive Coping Mode	
CHANGE PLAN: First Steps	
Healthy Adult Mode	

Translating Identified Problems into ST Concepts

In this exercise, you will translate your identified problem into ST concepts or language as a step in planning the interventions needed in Modules 8–12. Here are examples for our three therapists. If you like, go back to Chapter 3 to recall how they first described their problems.

 EXAMPLES: Julia's, Penny's, and Ian's Identified Problems Translated into ST Terms and Concepts

---

Julia: I have a tendency to avoid addressing my clients' emotion in therapy sessions, and this limits my effectiveness as a therapist. This situation activates my emotional inhibition schema, which triggers my Demanding Critic mode. Then my Vulnerable Child is triggered, and I end up feeling quite anxious and sad. In a session with a client, I might then flip to Detached Protector. This same pattern occurs when clients dismiss my interventions or cancel sessions. In those situations it is probably my Defectiveness/Shame schema that is activated, and if I am at home I flip into Detached Self-Soother and binge on chocolate.

In ST terms: I choose diminishing my Demanding Critic (thought level) and Detached Self-Soother (behavior level) modes as my identified problem for the workbook.

Penny: I struggle with times when clients in group ST don't do their homework. In viewing a recording of such a session, I could see that although my voice remained fairly neutral, the looks I was giving clients resembled that of a punitive teacher I'd had in high school. I also observed that I then gave the group an excessive homework assignment in that session. I recognize that my unrelenting standards schema is activated triggering my Perfectionistic Overcontroller mode. I continue working on this awareness as I realize that it interferes with my being a "good parent" for the group as well as setting realistic limits. I can do the same thing at home with my family. I think this mode of behavior leads to my adult children's reticence in discussing problems with me.

In ST terms, I choose to moderate my Perfectionistic Overcontroller as my identified problem.

Ian: I feel very anxious when I am preparing for supervision. I know that I can be quite defensive when I receive even constructive criticism, particularly from the senior supervisor. I hang on to the feeling that I know better and this gets communicated somehow. I notice that some colleagues seem to deliberately avoid doing role plays with me in training. I have been told that this behavior is an overcompensation for the Defectiveness/Shame schema, for which I have a high score on the YSQ. I am also very touchy in my personal relationship, and this causes tension and disconnection with my partner. My partner told me that she is beginning to avoid discussing problems with me, and it is damaging the relationship and causing her to withdraw from me.

In ST terms, I selected my Bully–Attack and Self-Aggrandizing behaviors in the Overcompensating Coping style as my identified problems, focusing on how they affect my personal and professional lives.

EXERCISE. My Identified Problems Translated into ST Terms

Self-Reflective Questions

What did you learn about yourself as a person and as a therapist from completing the Problem Analysis form? Were there any surprises?

_____

_____

_____

_____

_____

_____

_____

_____

_____

_____

_____

_____

_____

Were the exercises of Module 7 easy, difficult, or uncomfortable? What do you think accounts for any difficulty you experienced?

_____

_____

_____

_____

_____

_____

_____

_____

_____

_____

_____

_____

Are any schemas or modes activated for you? Which ones? What do you think caused the activation?

_____

_____

_____

_____

_____

_____

_____

_____

_____

_____

_____

_____

Was it useful to analyze your problem(s) in terms of schemas and modes? If so, will you use the Problem Analysis form with your clients in the future? How will you implement it?

_____

_____

_____

_____

_____

_____

_____

_____

_____

_____

_____

_____

What particularly stood out for you when considering your reaction to this first stage of the workbook, in which you identified a problematic area of your life, analyzed it, and set goals for change in terms of schemas and modes?

_____

_____

_____

_____

_____

_____

_____

_____

_____

_____

_____

_____

PART IV

The Beginning of Change
Mode Awareness and Mode Management

In **Modules 8 and 9** we focus on mode awareness and mode management for the Maladaptive Coping modes, and in **Modules 10 and 11**, the Dysfunctional Critic modes. We begin with mode awareness, which involves cognitive work to build a verbal and conceptual framework for later experiential work. Cognitive interventions are usually more familiar to clients than experiential work, and consequently they may feel safer. Cognitive interventions appeal to reasoning and engage the thinking, rational part of clients in challenging their schemas, recognizing schema modes, and strengthening access to their Healthy Adult mode. Awareness work is necessary, but not sufficient. It sets the stage for developing a mode management plan comprised of healthy actions to take in situations where schemas are activated. Mode awareness and mode management are components of ST that begin early in therapy and continue to be refined throughout treatment. **Module 12** focuses on strengthening your access to the Healthy Adult mode—the "director" of your action. In **Module 13** you will review your progress and your experience of the workbook to evaluate your readiness to continue to the experiential mode work.

The Steps to Change Dysfunctional Modes

1. Mode Awareness
   - Be aware of the Maladaptive Coping mode, first in retrospect and then with the "early warning signs" that it is beginning to operate (mode monitoring).
   - Make a decision about whether to change your Coping mode behavior by evaluating its effects (Pros and Cons exercise).
2. Mode Management
   - Learn healthier coping or ways to get underlying needs met (e.g., Safe-Place Image instead of avoidance).
   - Practice using the healthier coping behavior and record the results.

MODULE 8

Awareness of Your Maladaptive Coping Modes

> These exercises gave me new insights into how my Detached Protector works in relation to clients and in my life. My awareness definitely increased.
> —SP/SR participant

In Module 8 you are asked to summarize what you have learned about the effects related to your identified problem of the Coping modes you use and to make a Pros and Cons List regarding changing these behaviors.

Maladaptive Coping Mode Awareness Summary

Most of the problems our clients bring to therapy are due in part to the use of Maladaptive Coping modes in nonsurvival situations. Maladaptive Coping modes do not get the present need met, or if they do, they also have unwanted negative consequences.

 EXAMPLE: Ian's Maladaptive Coping Mode Awareness Summary

My overcompensating behavior that is either self-aggrandizing or attacking makes me feel important for a moment, but causes problems with my boss and alienates my peers. At home with my wife, it leads to her avoiding my company.

My identified problem is anxiety and dread, then self-aggrandizing behavior at home. I also have this problem at times in supervision and on the job, but I am currently most worried that I will alienate my wife if I continue these behaviors. I realize that when "Scared Ian" is activated by my Defectiveness/Shame schema, my immediate default response is an Overcompensating Coping mode like Self-Aggrandizer.

See Ian's Mode Awareness Summary Form on page 154.

IAN'S MODE AWARENESS SUMMARY FORM

Awareness summary for my _Overcompensating_____ mode	
Situations	My wife tells me I am not doing enough work around the house, or some other criticism. In ST supervision, I am told I left a step out of an intervention.
Early warning signs that this mode is triggered	I feel strong anxiety and a sense of dread too big for the present situation, then I become irritated and argumentative.
Physical sensations	Queasiness in the pit of my stomach
Feelings	I feel scared and hurt.
Thoughts	Why do they always have to one-up me by pointing out the things I don't do or that something is not perfect?
Related memory	Yes, it goes back to my perfectionistic father who was always picking at things I did. Nothing was good enough for him. I felt like I wasn't good enough for him. I was also punished severely for any mistake—like forgetting to take the garbage out the minute it was full.
Schema activated	Defectiveness/Shame
Survival function of the mode	If I did not argue. I felt I would be crushed—I would be agreeing that I was a bad kid.
What **need** is present?	Validation, acknowledgment, acceptance
Usual action taken	I tell the person that he or she is wrong and start listing what a good husband (psychotherapist) I am. I tell my wife how fortunate she is to have me, and sometimes I say something to hurt her feelings or to put her down.
Does my action get the need met?	No, my wife gets mad and leaves the room, making a sarcastic comment. My supervisor elaborates on why he is correct and I am wrong and points out my mode activation.
Do I flip into another mode?	Detached Protector: Sometimes I detach in response to their comments or I leave the situation showing that I am angry.

 EXERCISE. My Maladaptive Coping Mode Awareness Summary

Now select the Maladaptive Coping mode you noted as related to your identified problem and complete the blank Mode Awareness Summary Form on page 155.

MY MODE AWARENESS SUMMARY FORM

Awareness summary for my _____ mode	
Situations	
Early warning signs that this mode is triggered	
Physical sensations	
Feelings	
Thoughts	
Related memory	
Schema activated	
Survival function of the mode	
What **need** is present?	
Usual action taken	
Does my action get the need met?	
Do I flip into another mode?	

From *Experiencing Schema Therapy from the Inside Out: A Self-Practice/Self-Reflection Workbook for Therapists* by Joan M. Farrell and Ida A. Shaw. Copyright © 2018 The Guilford Press. Permission to photocopy this form is granted to purchasers of this book for personal use only (see copyright page for details). Purchasers can download additional copies of this form (see the box at the end of the table of contents).

A Pros and Cons List for Changing Maladaptive Coping Modes

The next step is to use your awareness of your needs in the present and the effect of your old survival coping behavior to decide about whether to change the frequency or intensity of your Maladaptive Coping mode behavior. This decision is a crucial step in treatment. Your Coping modes helped you to survive difficult and painful situations in your past, particularly in childhood. This is one reason why they may have so much power over you now. The idea of changing your Maladaptive Coping mode will feel very vulnerable and scary because the Vulnerable Child mode is involved, bringing up memories and strong feelings from childhood experiences. The Pros and Cons List provides a current assessment of your Coping mode's function. The next step is to identify an alternative Healthy Adult mode behavior that could better meet your adult needs.

Ian's Pros and Cons List is illustrated beginning below. We ask clients to keep this analysis as a reference. We inevitably need to refer to it when they are in the grip of a Maladaptive Coping mode and don't remember why they decided to do the difficult work of changing it. You can also use it for reference, as we therapists are subject to the same pull back to what is familiar as our clients are.

 IAN'S PROS AND CONS LIST

Pros and Cons for keeping the <u>Self-Aggrandizing</u> mode at its current intensity		
From past situations in which I used the old Coping mode behavior	PROS: Reasons **not to change**	CONS: Reasons **to change**
	As a child, bragging about my accomplishments helped me feel less defective. It let people know how good I was.	My father would say even more mean things to "cut me down to size," he said. Peers made fun of my bragging.
From situations in the last 3 months in which I used old Coping mode behavior	I feel powerful when I am self-aggrandizing. I don't have to feel inferior or defective. It temporarily quiets my self-critical voice.	My wife says she is tired of my bragging and one-upping her. She feels embarrassed when I brag in public. My coworkers make fun of me behind my back.
What need of the Vulnerable Child mode underlies the Maladaptive Coping mode?	Acceptance, validation, to feel lovable	
Does the old Coping mode behavior meet the need?	No, it usually leads to rejection.	

Are there results from the Coping mode that I don't like? Does it damage my relationships?	I feel guilty later for what I have said to my wife. Yes, it drives my wife away and is creating unwanted distance between us.
Should I change my old Coping mode behavior?	YES—I could approach my need more effectively using skills I have acquired as a therapist.
Does my usual **action get my need met?**	No—my wife has told me that she feels she cannot discuss any problems with me and is disgusted and embarrassed that I am such a braggart.
What is my decision regarding change?	The Cons clearly outweigh the Pros, so I will work to change these old Coping behaviors.

EXERCISE. My Pros and Cons List

Now make a Pros and Cons List and need analysis for yourself using the form beginning below. There are prompts in the form to stimulate your thinking, but these are not meant to limit the list to those aspects. Feel free to add your own, as we tell clients to do.

MY PROS AND CONS LIST

Pros and Cons for keeping the _____ mode at its current intensity		
From past situations in which I used the old Coping mode behavior	PROS: Reasons **not to change**	CONS: Reasons **to change**
From situations in the last 3 months in which I used old Coping mode behavior		
What need of the Vulnerable Child mode underlies the Maladaptive Coping mode?		
Does the old Coping mode behavior meet the need?		

Are there results from the Coping mode that I don't like? Does it damage my relationships?	
Should I change my old Coping mode behavior?	
Does my usual **action get my need met?**	
What is my decision regarding change?	

 ASSIGNMENT

Add to your Mode Awareness Summary Form throughout the week as you notice any Maladaptive Coping mode behavior.

Self-Reflective Questions

Were you able to identify times when you responded to a situation, thought, or feeling with a Coping mode? If so, how did it feel to be aware of this?

_____

_____

_____

_____

_____

_____

_____

_____

_____

_____

_____

_____

_____

What were your thoughts and feelings after completing the Pros and Cons List about possibly making some changes? Was it helpful? If so, in what manner? Were there any surprises?

_____

_____

_____

_____

_____

_____

_____

_____

_____

_____

_____

_____

What are the key things you have learned about yourself during this module that you would like to remember?

_____

_____

_____

_____

_____

_____

_____

_____

_____

_____

_____

_____

Are there any particular clients or people who routinely trigger your Coping modes? Can you understand why this may be happening? What do you want to do differently in responding to them?

_____

_____

_____

_____

_____

_____

_____

_____

_____

_____

_____

_____

_____

Think about one of your most difficult clients. Is there anything in this module that might explain why he or she has struggled to engage with or benefit from treatment? How might your awareness of your own Coping modes affect your attitude and/or behavior about that client?

_____

_____

_____

_____

_____

_____

_____

_____

_____

_____

_____

_____

_____

A Management Plan
for Your Maladaptive Coping Modes

It is interesting that I struggle with the same modes in my work and personal life.
I realized that I either avoid attending to them with clients or I get stuck there.
This module helped me realize that this is something I really need to work on.
—SP/SR participant

In Module 9 you will use your Awareness Summary for your default Coping mode to formulate a plan for behavioral pattern-breaking work. We refer to this as a Mode Management Plan, and you will develop one for each of your main dysfunctional modes. These plans spell out specifically the change work needed to meet the goals you set for these modes.

Notes. Mode Management Plans are one of the main components of ST, as described in Chapter 2. They act as plans for the behavioral pattern-breaking stage, an essential component of change in ST. The first step in decreasing Maladaptive Coping mode actions was the self-monitoring you did using the Self-Monitoring Circle form of Module 6. In order to have a choice about what kind of action to take, you need to *notice* the activation of a schema or the beginning of a Maladaptive Coping mode being triggered. To begin with, you may only notice this triggering in retrospect. The Coping mode is automatic; it does not seem to be a conscious choice. There are four basic choices in every situation: fight, flight, freeze, or access the Healthy Adult mode. We have a choice once we become aware of the triggering of a dysfunctional mode before any action is taken. Behavior change starts in sessions in the context of the therapy relationship or in mode dialogues or mode role plays and then moves to the outside world. This stage begins when you are aware of a schema-driven dysfunctional mode being triggered and are able to choose a healthier response that will get your needs met. It is important during this stage to have a written plan, to continue to collect evidence about the improved outcome of the new strategies, and to practice and fine-tune them.

Developing a Mode Management Plan

The first step in formulating a plan to change your automatic Coping mode behavior is to identify what Healthy Adult action you could take that would better meet your identified need. Ian's first step is described in the form below.

 IAN'S MODE MANAGEMENT PLAN, STEP 1

Need	Validation	
What else could I do to try to meet this need?	I could tell my wife that I need more validation for my accomplishments and to hear that I am doing a good job.	
What are the pros and cons of the new alternative?	Pro: She would probably give me what I ask for.	Con: I would be vulnerable in saying what I need. Vulnerability is weakness, and it is dangerous.
Results of trying the Healthy Adult behavior		
Try the new behavior and record the result here.	Tried it, and it wasn't too scary. I felt vulnerable and a bit frightened when I began talking to her. She gave me some nice compliments, and I felt warm and secure, closer to her.	

 EXERCISE. My Mode Management Plan, Step 1

Complete the chart on page 164 with the Healthy Adult behavior that could meet the need you identified in the **My Maladaptive Coping Mode Awareness Summary** exercise in Module 8.

MY MODE MANAGEMENT PLAN, STEP 1

Need	Validation	
What else could I do to try to meet this need?		
What are the pros and cons of the new alternative?		
Results of trying the Healthy Adult behavior		
Try the new behavior and record the result here.		

From *Experiencing Schema Therapy from the Inside Out: A Self-Practice/Self-Reflection Workbook for Therapists* by Joan M. Farrell and Ida A. Shaw. Copyright © 2018 The Guilford Press. Permission to photocopy this form is granted to purchasers of this book for personal use only (see copyright page for details). Purchasers can download additional copies of this form (see the box at the end of the table of contents).

Fine-Tuning Your Mode Management Plan

The next step is to develop a more elaborated Mode Management Plan based upon your experience in trying out various healthy behaviors to meet the need you identified in the previous exercise. Mode management is discussed in detail in Chapter 2. Julia's completed Maladaptive Coping Mode Management Plan appears beginning below.

 JULIA'S MALADAPTIVE COPING MODE MANAGEMENT PLAN

My Mode Management Plan for <u>Detached Protector</u> (fill in the Maladaptive Coping mode)	
Which EMS triggers this mode?	Defectiveness/Shame
What need is involved?	To feel competent and acceptable, not defective.
How could I get the need met in a healthy way?	If I can set the limits needed when my clients are in the Bully–Attack mode, I will be able to stay present and respond like a competent therapist.

What mode flip might interfere with healthy action?	If I listen to my Demanding Critic, who says, "You always get it wrong, so don't even try."
Reality check: What are the objective facts of this situation?	Many of my peers said they also have difficulty with the Bully–Attack mode and wanted to practice. I did not feel as defective and incompetent hearing that. I was able to set limits effectively in peer supervision, and my colleagues gave me positive feedback.
How can I use my awareness of the Maladaptive Coping mode to stop and make a choice?	When I noticed feeling a little spacey, I grounded myself by feeling my feet on the floor and breathing into my center. That allowed me to be in my Healthy Adult mode. In that mode I can take healthy actions to get my needs met.
How could my Healthy Adult mode challenge the Critic's message?	I can remind myself that if I don't try, I will never succeed or feel competent. It is not a terrible thing to try and fail. It does not make me incompetent because I am not perfect. When I practiced with peers, I improved. I can do it.
What was the result and was my need met?	The session went better and, yes, my need to feel more competent was met.
What new message can I use as an "antidote" against the Critic mode?	I am not defective and worthless, I am a beginner schema therapist, and I need practice.

Notes. You will notice that Julia and Ian are working with the same EMS—Defectiveness/Shame—which is a very common core schema. However, we have seen that Ian's default coping style is Overcompensating and his usual Coping modes are Self-Aggrandizing or Bully–Attack, whereas Julia's default coping style is Avoidance and her usual Coping modes are Detached Protector or Detached Self-Soother.

EXERCISE. My Maladaptive Coping Mode Management Plan

Now you will develop a Mode Management Plan for yourself for the Maladaptive Coping mode that is most involved in your identified problem (see form on p. 166).

MY MALADAPTIVE COPING MODE MANAGEMENT PLAN

My Mode Management Plan for _____ (fill in the Maladaptive Coping mode)	
Which EMS triggers this mode?	
What need is involved?	
How could I get the need met in a healthy way?	
What mode flip might interfere with healthy action?	
Reality check: What are the objective facts of this situation?	
How can I use my awareness of the Maladaptive Coping mode to stop and make a choice?	
How could my Healthy Adult mode challenge the Critic's message?	
What was the result and was my need met?	
What new message can I use as an "antidote" against the Critic mode?	

Notes. We do not want to suggest that changing old coping behavior, which began as a survival strategy in childhood when core needs were not met, is a simple or easy thing to accomplish. Awareness of the Coping mode being used and the fact that it does not get your current needs met provides motivation to make these changes. As you can see in the example given, Julia ran into interference from her Critic mode, which also had to be addressed. This interference happens very frequently and is another of the ways in which clients and therapists can get stuck. Another possibility is that the Vulnerable Child's fear is so great that it prevents taking the risk of using a new behavior. In either case, the interfering mode must be addressed before behavior change can take hold. The Dysfunctional Critic mode is addressed in the next module. Some suggestions to use for diminishing the Critic's power are given in Julia's example below.

JULIA'S SUMMARY OF HER MODE MANAGEMENT PLAN RESULTS

Actions taken	Before I went into a session with a client who has a strong Bully-Attack mode, I accessed my Safe-Place Image for Little Julia and connected with my Healthy Adult mode by using the Physical Grounding exercises in Module 1.
Results	I could stay present and set a limit more effectively than usual.
Was my NEED met?	Yes, I felt good about the session and more competent. I did not allow the client to berate me, and I protected Little Julia effectively.
Healthy Adult message to take from this	When I connect with my Healthy Adult mode, I am able to implement ST interventions competently for the client and for myself.

 EXERCISE. My Summary of My Mode Management Plan Results

In the form on page 168, you will summarize what you have learned from using your Mode Management Plan by formulating a Healthy Adult message.

MY SUMMARY OF MY MODE MANAGEMENT PLAN RESULTS

Actions taken	
Results	
Was my NEED met?	
Healthy Adult message to take from this	

ASSIGNMENT

Record the results of using your Mode Management Plan over the next week.

Healthy Adult mode actions
Results

Was my underlying need met?

Cognitive antidote: Summarize these positive experiences into a new message and record it here.

From your results over these 2 weeks, you may want to fine-tune your Mode Management Plan so that it fits you even better.

Self-Reflective Questions

What was helpful about the Mode Management Plan exercise?

_____

_____

_____

_____

_____

_____

_____

_____

_____

_____

_____

_____

_____

Consider again the difficult client about whom you thought after Module 8. If you are able to modify your behavior when a Coping mode is triggered, how will it alter your attitude about, and approach to, this client?

_____

_____

_____

_____

_____

_____

_____

_____

_____

_____

_____

_____

Answer the next questions after you complete the assignment for Module 9.

Did you use your Mode Management Plan? What did you notice about the experience of carrying out this plan?

_____

_____

_____

_____

_____

_____

_____

_____

_____

_____

_____

_____

_____

If yes, what was the result? Was your underlying need met?

_____

_____

_____

_____

_____

_____

_____

_____

_____

_____

_____

_____

_____

_____

If no, what interfered? Was a schema activated? A mode triggered?

_____

_____

_____

_____

_____

_____

_____

_____

_____

_____

_____

Now that you have experienced having an ST homework assignment, does it give you any new insight regarding your clients' experiences with receiving and completing therapy assignments?

_____

_____

_____

_____

_____

_____

_____

_____

_____

_____

_____

_____

Awareness of
Your Dysfunctional Critic Modes

> In this exercise, I saw how my Demanding Critic mode
> expects results from clients and pushes them. This was
> very helpful both for me as a therapist and as a person.
> —SP/SR participant

The next category of modes, which are involved in most psychological problems, is the Dysfunctional Critic mode. In previous modules, you identified your Dysfunctional Critic mode and how it is related to your identified problem. Module 10 focuses on awareness of the content of your Dysfunctional Critic mode—the distorted and exaggerated negative messages and rules that come to mind in this mode. You will summarize what you know about your version of the Critic on a Mode Awareness Summary Form.

Notes. Our early experience of the world comes from the way our parents or caregivers treat us and respond to us. Young children define the world in terms of themselves. In this normal stage of development, we feel that the world revolves around us, our needs are all that exist, and everything that happens is because of us. An example is when kids blame themselves for their parents' divorce. When parents are punitive and critical, children feel that they are "bad" and "the problem." Sometimes unhealthy caregivers tell kids children, for example, "I wouldn't lose my temper and hit you if you weren't such a bad kid." An extreme example occurs in sexual abuse where perpetrators tell the children that they "are to blame" because *they* "wanted it," etc. Children are never to blame for abuse! As children, we also internalize what the important people around us say about us and how they describe us. These statements become part of our internal dialogue and self-concept, whether they are accurate or not. They are reinforced over time by the selective internalization of statements that confirm them, and they become our core beliefs about ourselves, the world, and other people. We accept them as true and, even as adults, do not check their accuracy.

The Dysfunctional Critic modes (presented in Chapter 2) store the negative messages that we take away from experiences in childhood and adolescence in which our core needs were not met. These messages become core beliefs, the cognitive aspect of schemas. Ella's experience in the thunderstorm story of Module 4 (p. 102) is an example of how a child who does not have her need for safety and comfort met feels that her feelings and needs were wrong and consequently that she is "wrong or bad in some way." Ella also took away the message or belief that she was "on her own, no help was available." Messages like these are not necessarily verbalized, but rather they represent the child or adolescent's perception of what his or her experience meant. The thoughts that run through a person's mind when Dysfunctional Critic modes are triggered reflect such negative core beliefs. We may or may not recall the specific memories of origin for our Critic messages.

Young et al. (2003) conceptualized this selective negative internalization as the Dysfunctional Parent modes, which we have renamed Dysfunctional Critic (presented in Chapter 2). These modes can represent one or both parents' or early caregiver's anger, neglect, abuse, unrelenting standards; a bully or negative peer group from childhood or adolescence (e.g., labels such as "fatty," "queer," "uncool"); or negative feedback or demands from coaches and teachers. We refer to these dysfunctional modes as Critic modes rather than Dysfunctional Parent modes because they are usually an amalgam of negative messages not always from parents and not necessarily intended. In addition, many clients are still living with parents with whom they need to interact in a healthy manner, and we feel this changed label avoids unnecessarily triggering family loyalty responses in our clients. It is important to remind clients that identifying a "Critic" mode does not mean that there was nothing good about their parents or that they should not have positive feelings toward them. In some cases, particularly for clients with BPD and/or complex trauma, a parent(s) is the primary source of the Critic mode and the client may choose to label their Critic as a Punitive or Demanding Parent. We leave the choice up to each client.

⚒ EXERCISE. Increasing Your Awareness of the Dysfunctional Critic Mode

The Critic sees the world through a filter of distortions based upon your schemas; thus little or no disconfirming evidence is collected. Awareness of a Dysfunctional Critic mode operating requires that you learn to recognize the critical, punishing, or demanding messages that automatically occur in your thoughts. Examples of some Critic messages and the EMS they reflect:

- "You are just not likable." (Defectiveness/Shame EMS)
- "You must always put everyone else's need before your own." (Self-Sacrifice EMS)
- "You must look and be perfect." (Unrelenting Standards EMS)
- "You will never accomplish enough to be good." (Failure EMS)
- "You are such a whiner, always saying you are sad and lonely" (Emotional Inhibition EMS)

Young et al. (2003) distinguished two types of Critic: one is Punitive, focusing on how rules are enforced, and the other Demanding, focusing on the standards and rules themselves, not their enforcement. The Dysfunctional Critic may be Punitive or Demanding or both Punitive and Demanding. In the Punitive Critic mode, you blame and/or punish yourself for normal needs that you were not allowed to express. You may describe yourself as "bad," "worthless," "stupid," "a loser," or some other pejorative term. The Punitive Critic mode is one of the modes in which clients with BPD self-injure. In the Demanding Critic mode, you are pushed to high achievement by the idea that any accomplishment could always be "better" and that mistakes, even small ones, are unacceptable. In this mode you feel that you must be perfect so you strive for high status, keep everything in order, act efficiently, and avoid wasting any time. You feel it is wrong to express feelings or to act spontaneously. Many subtypes are possible: for example, the Cynic, the Pessimist, the Nagger, and the Dictator. It is important to identify your own version, name it in a meaningful way for you, and develop awareness of when it is triggered and what faulty messages come with it.

 EXAMPLE: Julia's Awareness of Her Dysfunctional Critic mode

I have a strong Unrelenting Standards schema from childhood experiences with a perfectionistic mother who thought that whatever I did could always be done better. I almost never received positive feedback on my performance, so I also developed a Defectiveness/Shame EMS. When either (or both) of these schemas is activated, my Demanding and Punitive Critic mode is triggered. In this mode, I berate myself for not doing more—for example, not finding the "perfect" intervention to use with a difficult client. Although the words were never spoken, I experienced the implicit message from my mother that if I am not perfect, I would have no worth and I would be "stupid." So, whenever I make a mistake, the message that comes to mind automatically is "You stupid idiot!" I feel queasy in my stomach with a sense of dread, and I remember times when I felt the disappointment of my mother. In ST terms, I have learned that I flip from my Critic mode to my Vulnerable Child, in which I feel sad, rejected, and unloved. In the Child mode, I remember other experiences in which only perfection counted— like being criticized in front of my class at school when I received a 99 on an algebra test because of a mistake in addition. It was the highest mark in the class, but not good enough for me, "Sister Anne's star pupil." She made that very clear to everyone.

When I can stand the pain of my Child no longer, a Coping mode takes over to allow escape. For me this is either the Perfectionistic Overcontroller mode (Overcompensating style) or the Detached Protector (Avoidant style). [These modes are described in Chapter 2.] The former leads to relentless reading and workshop attending, as one "can never know enough," and the latter leads to detaching and not being emotionally present in psychotherapy sessions with challenging clients. My Perfectionistic Overcontroller leaves little time for interpersonal relationships or pleasurable activities—I am "all work"—and the lack of genuine presence when I am in Detached Protector limits how effective I can be with my clients.

The goal of ST for the Dysfunctional Critic modes is to diminish their power over you and their control over your actions. Psychotherapists often have a strong Demanding

Critic mode, triggered by EMS frequently found in this group—Unrelenting Standards and/or Self-Sacrifice.

Identifying Your Dysfunctional Critic's Messages

The first step in changing your Critic is to become aware of its messages. As adults we are usually not conscious of, and therefore we do not challenge, our Critic's messages. They are our core beliefs; we accept them as truth. You can increase your awareness by identifying your thoughts in situations in which you feel self-critical, blaming, or punitive. This exercise asks you to record your Critic's messages.

 EXAMPLE: Penny's Dysfunctional Critic's Messages

Penny's messages are similar to Julia's. They are an example of how the Dysfunctional Critic mode can generate rules about how to be safe in the world that limit getting your adult needs met.

---

1. My main Punitive/Demanding message:

You have made another mistake—you are such an idiot.

You need to work harder and longer; your work could be better.

2. Where did it come from? Who does it sound like?

No one ever said those words to me, but I constructed them from the disgust I saw in my mother and teachers whenever I made a mistake or was less than perfect.

3. Which message is related to your identified problem?

You need to work harder and longer; your work could be better.

 EXAMPLE: Ian's Dysfunctional Critic's Message

Ian has slightly different Critic message related to expressing his feelings.

---

1. My main Punitive or Demanding Critic message:

The rule is, never let anyone see you as hurt. It makes you weak, and others will take advantage and hurt you more. Men should never be weak and never show hurt feelings.

2. Where did it come from? Who does it sound like?

It came from my father. He told me this often and proved it by hurting me more whenever I cried as a child. I learned quickly to keep a "stiff upper lip" with him.

3. Which message is related to your identified problem?

The one about never showing hurt feelings. Instead, whenever I feel criticized, I seem to jump automatically to attacking the person involved to protect myself.

EXERCISE. My Dysfunctional Critic's Message

Now fill in this information for your Dysfunctional Critic mode message related to your identified problem.

---

1. **My main Punitive/Demanding message:**

2. **Where did it come from? Who does it sound like?**

3. **Which message is related to your identified problem?**

The Dysfunctional Critic Mode Awareness Summary

As with the other modes, the first step toward change is developing an understanding of what your experience of a mode is and then noticing early warning signs that the mode has been triggered. The earlier you can recognize the Critic, the more effective your Healthy Adult mode can be in challenging its messages and effects. Julia completed the Dysfunctional Critic Mode Awareness Summary form as illustrated beginning below.

 JULIA'S DYSFUNCTIONAL CRITIC MODE AWARENESS SUMMARY

Situations	When I have to explain an ST experiential exercise like imagery rescripting and my client reacts like I am not making any sense.

Early warning signs that this mode is triggered	The first thing I notice is the look of confusion on my client's face.
Physical sensations	I feel queasy in my stomach.
Feelings	I feel anxious and frightened.
Thoughts (my critic's message)	I have the thought "You are just not good enough to be a schema therapist. You are too stupid and never get it right."
Related memory	I remember telling Grandma in front of my mother about a problem with our neighbor. Grandma got mad at Mother, and Mom yelled at me the way home saying that I had explained it all wrong and caused a misunderstanding between them. She said I that if I could not be clear, I should just keep my mouth shut.
Schema(s) activated	Defectiveness/Shame, Unrelenting Standards
Survival function of the mode	I am not sure my Critic has a survival function—maybe it protected me in a sense because it said "Don't bother trying, you won't do it right"—so I was never disappointed, but I generally kept quiet and was not recognized in class or paid attention to at home.
What need is present?	Validation, acceptance just as I am, imperfect.
Usual action taken	I usually stay up late rereading the ST material to be able to explain concepts better.
Does my action get the need met?	No. I am tired in the morning, sleepy in client sessions, and am more likely to be anxious and make a bigger muddle of my explanations.
Do I flip into another mode?	Detached Protector. I go through the motions in sessions, watching the clock until the session time is up.

 EXERCISE. My Dysfunctional Critic Mode Awareness Summary

Now name your Critic mode and complete the Awareness Summary form on pages 180–181 for your experience.

MY DYSFUNCTIONAL CRITIC MODE AWARENESS SUMMARY

Situations	
Early warning signs that this mode is triggered	
Physical sensations	
Feelings	
Thoughts (my critic's message)	
Related memory	
Schema(s) activated	
Survival function of the mode	
What **need** is present?	
Usual action taken	
Does my action get the need met?	
Do I flip into another mode?	

ASSIGNMENT

Over the next week or until you begin Module 11, add anything else you notice about your experience of the Critic mode to your Awareness Summary. In Module 11 we will work on challenging the Critic's messages. For now, we collect those messages as part of developing awareness of when the Critic mode is operating.

Self-Reflective Questions

How did you experience the process of identifying your Punitive or Demanding Critic mode messages or rules? Did you have any emotional, behavioral, bodily, or cognitive responses? Any surprises or difficulties?

_____

_____

_____

_____

_____

_____

_____

_____

_____

_____

_____

_____

Are the messages or rules you identified as your Critic mode related to your identified problem? If so, how?

_____

_____

_____

_____

_____

_____

_____

_____

_____

_____

_____

_____

Do you see any connections between the Critic's messages for your therapist self versus your personal self? How do you understand these connections? What are the implications?

_____

_____

_____

_____

_____

_____

_____

_____

_____

_____

_____

_____

_____

Did you notice any cultural or religious/spiritual influences on your Critic? Can you describe these and comment on how influential they might have been.

_____

_____

_____

_____

_____

_____

_____

_____

_____

_____

_____

Bring to mind a client with whom you feel stuck. Does the experience of noticing your own Dysfunctional Critic mode shed different light on understanding him or her?

_____

_____

_____

_____

_____

_____

_____

_____

_____

_____

_____

_____

_____

How easy or difficult was it for you to identify the sources (person, people, experiences, etc.) of your Dysfunctional Critic? Did your experience from the "inside out" add anything to your understanding of this process for clients? Will you do anything differently with your clients based upon your experience?

_____

_____

_____

_____

_____

_____

_____

_____

_____

_____

_____

_____

_____

MODULE 11

A Management Plan
for Your Dysfunctional Critic Modes

> I realized from the exercises for the Critic mode that I still have
> some work to do. I believe as a therapist that it is invaluable to
> take the time to work on my own issues and grow as a person.
> —SP/SR participant

In this module 11 you will develop *Cognitive Antidotes* to challenge your Dysfunctional Critic ode and a Mode Management Plan for *Behavioral Antidotes* for the Critic. *Experiential Antidotes* will be developed in Module 18.

Notes. For clients at the beginning of ST, the idea that core beliefs are the result of our particular childhood experiences of needs not being met is an alien concept. The ideas that schemas distort our view, acting as a filter for new information and experience, and bias our interpretation of events are all new to them. We see "all-or-none" dichotomous thinking as a main cognitive distortion of the Critic mode. The Critic's message is some version of "Either you are perfect, brilliant, beautiful, etc., or worthless, stupid, unappealing, etc." In people with personality disorders, these messages reflect negative core beliefs and are extremely rigid and entrenched. Core beliefs are accepted as "facts" and determine the way we view the world, ourselves, and other people. It is important to create doubt about these negative core beliefs in order to change them. In ST, we begin by challenging them at the cognitive level, as clients are usually more familiar with this approach. If this should not be the case with you or your client. just reverse the order of approach. This is an example of the flexibility of ST in matching what fits best for the client. ST goes on to address the emotional level with interventions that provide corrective emotional experiences that contradict the negative core belief at the emotional level. This level of experience is addressed in Module 18 and added to the Mode Management

Plan at that time. Ultimately, we also need to address the actions that result from these negative core beliefs via behavioral pattern-breaking antidotes. A strength of ST is this comprehensive approach to change at all three aspects of experience.

The Dysfunctional Critic modes operate primarily at the cognitive level, but can trigger the emotions of the Vulnerable Child and/or the actions of the Maladaptive Coping modes. This kind of chain of triggering is often referred to as "mode flipping." It is discussed in Chapter 2 on page 18 and shown in Figure 2.2 (p. 19). An example for Julia is presented below.

 EXAMPLE: Julia's Mode Flipping in Response to Her Demanding Critic

Aspect of experience		Mode triggered
Cognition	*You never work hard enough. You need at least four more hours on this report. You could do better.*	**Dysfunctional Critic** *Slave driver*
Emotion	*Anxiety, shame*	**Vulnerable Child** *Little Julia*
	Anger	**Angry Child** *Pissed-off Julia*
Behavior	*I stop working, with the report unfinished. I watch reality TV the rest of the night and stuff myself with popcorn.*	**Detached Self-Soother** *Who cares—I'm bored Julia*

Developing Cognitive Antidotes

The steps of a developing an antidote for the cognitive aspect of your Dysfunctional Critic mode are:

1. Recognize the automatic thoughts that stem from your negative core beliefs.
2. Identify any cognitive distortions present.
3. Consider healthy alternatives. Write them down or record them on your smartphone/tablet so you will have easy access to them.
4. If you can't come up with a Healthy Adult mode alternative, ask someone you trust for help.

Cognitive Antidotes are statements that you can make to yourself that contradict the belief or thinking part of the mode. For example, if you have a harsh Critic mode and have the automatic thought "You stupid idiot" any time you make a mistake, a Cognitive Antidote could be a challenging statement in which you also believe to some degree. An example would be "Making a mistake does not make me an idiot; making a mistake just shows that I am human. I can learn from this." This example reframes the mistake in a healthier perspective—the perspective of the Healthy Adult mode. Some mistakes do have consequences and may affect our relationships or work. If you take the Healthy Adult mode attitude of "Learn from mistakes," rather than flipping into the Punitive Critic and disparaging yourself, while taking responsibility for any negative fall-out, you will be more effective and able to improve. Psychotherapists have these critical messages also. Both of us can recognize our Critic's messages and continue to work on reducing their effects.

 EXAMPLE: Penny's Cognitive Antidote for the Dysfunctional Critic Mode

---

My thoughts/Critic's message

You never work hard enough. You need at least 4 more hours on this report. You could do better.

Evidence that supports the message

I might do better if I work even longer, but then I will be exhausted tomorrow and not function well.

Evidence that contradicts or qualifies the message

I have worked long and hard enough on this report. It is not my PhD thesis; it is more than good enough for its purpose. Working longer is not necessarily better. There is a point of diminishing return.

What I can say to contradict the Critic's message = Cognitive Antidote

I am good at writing reports, and this one is good enough. I need my sleep also to feel healthy tomorrow.

The last two statements comprise a "Cognitive Antidote" for the Dysfunctional Critic mode. Now fill in your main Critic message related to your identified problem and develop a Cognitive Antidote.

 EXERCISE. My Cognitive Antidote for the Dysfunctional Critic Mode

---

My thoughts/Critic's message

Evidence that supports the message

Evidence that contradicts or qualifies the message

> **What I can say to contradict the Critic's message = Cognitive Antidote**

Behavioral Pattern-Breaking Antidotes

It is also important to consider the automatic behaviors that occur when you are in Dysfunctional Critic modes. In the ST model, these behaviors are seen as part of the Maladaptive Coping modes. A behavioral pattern-breaking antidote consists of taking a healthy action to get your underlying need met instead of following the rule of your Critic. The next step in diminishing the power of your Dysfunctional Critic mode is formulating a Mode Management Plan. This is a plan for how you will use the cognitive and behavioral antidotes you developed to meet the goal for the Critic mode from your Problem Analysis form of Module 7. An example from Julia is presented in the Mode Management Plan beginning below. You will add an Experiential Antidote to the plan in Module 18.

 JULIA'S DYSFUNCTIONAL CRITIC MODE MANAGEMENT PLAN

Activating situation	It is 9 p.m. and I have a report due tomorrow that I need to finish.
Schemas activated	Unrelenting Standards
Mode triggered	Detached Self-Soother
Emotions	Anxious, worrying
What do you need?	More than just work—nourishment and a break.
Old coping mode action	I stop working with the report unfinished, I watch reality TV the rest of the night, and stuff myself with popcorn.
Need met?	No. It is after midnight, the report is not finished, and I feel uncomfortably stuffed.
How could I fight my Critic and meet my needs?	
Cognitive Antidote	I can tell myself "What you have done so far is good enough for now. You can finish up after dinner."
Behavioral Antidote	I can ignore my Critic and take a 45-minute break and eat dinner.

Experiential Antidote	[Added in Module 18]
Result	I finish up the report in half an hour and get to bed by 11 p.m.

✍️ **EXERCISE.** My Dysfunctional Critic Mode Management Plan

Below, work on your Dysfunctional Critic Mode Management Plan related to your identified problem.

MY DYSFUNCTIONAL CRITIC MODE MANAGEMENT PLAN

Activating situation	
Schemas activated	
Mode triggered	
Emotions	
What do you need?	
Old coping mode action	
Need met?	
How could I fight my Critic and meet my needs?	
Cognitive Antidote	
Behavioral Antidote	
Experiential Antidote	[Added in Module 18]
Result	

ASSIGNMENT

Put your Dysfunctional Critic Mode Management Plan in a place where you will see it frequently (about once a day, not constantly). Try to use it a few times per week while we are on Module 11. Record the results in the chart below.

New action (Healthy Adult mode)	Was my need met?

Self-Reflective Questions

What did you identify as the triggers of your Critic mode?

_____

_____

_____

_____

_____

_____

_____

_____

_____

_____

What new messages were you able to develop to use as Cognitive Antidotes? In considering these messages, what feelings, thoughts, or sensations are you aware of?

_____

_____

_____

_____

_____

_____

_____

_____

_____

_____

_____

_____

What was it like to construct a new Good Parent message? Do you believe the new message from your head (cognitive knowing) versus from your heart (felt sense)? What sense do you make of it if there is a conflict?

_____

_____

_____

_____

_____

_____

_____

_____

_____

_____

_____

_____

_____

In your work with the Dysfunctional Critic modes, which exercises were the most helpful in adding to your understanding of yourself?

_____

_____

_____

_____

_____

_____

_____

_____

_____

_____

_____

_____

Which exercises were least helpful?

_____

_____

_____

_____

_____

_____

_____

_____

_____

_____

_____

_____

Which exercises do you see using with clients you are working with now?

_____

_____

_____

_____

_____

_____

_____

_____

_____

_____

What did you notice about your experience of using your Mode Management Plan? Was there anything that surprised you?

_____

_____

_____

_____

_____

_____

_____

_____

_____

_____

Strengthening Your Healthy Adult Mode

I was surprised by the impact an ST flashcard for my Vulnerable Child had when I flipped for a moment when a client in the Bully–Attack mode was yelling at me. Usually when I was triggered like that, I would go into Detached Protector, but this time I reached my Healthy Adult and set the necessary limit with the client.
—SP/SR participant

The overarching goal of ST is to develop and strengthen the Healthy Adult mode of a person so that he or she is able to get the needs that underlie the Dysfunctional modes met in a healthy manner. In Module 12 we ask you to collect information about your Healthy Adult mode and explore ways to access it.

Notes. A childhood environment where love, support, encouragement, validation, and consistency are provided and experienced promotes the development of a strong Healthy Adult mode. Most people with a psychiatric disorder did not have such a childhood environment and do not have a strong Healthy Adult or Happy Child mode. Fortunately, the healthy modes can be strengthened in ST. Positive changes posttreatment on the SMI support this assertion (Farrell et al., 2014).

In the Healthy Adult mode, we are able to balance needs and responsibilities so that we can enjoy life but also have fulfilling work. From the Healthy Adult mode we take on adult functions like work, parenting, and other duties and pursue pleasurable activities such as sexuality, intellectual and cultural interests, and sports. The Healthy Adult mode can be thought of as the director of the Dysfunctional modes. When you are in the Healthy Adult mode:

- You support, validate, and meet the needs of your Vulnerable Child mode.
- You set limits for your Angry and impulsive Child mode, but hear the need.
- You find and develop your Happy Child mode.

- You fight your Dysfunctional Critic modes.
- You replace your Maladaptive Coping modes with healthy coping strategies.

The Healthy Adult mode has "Good Parent" skills of varying strength. What we refer to as the Good Parent aspect of the Healthy Adult consists of comforting and soothing skills that we have taken in or internalized from healthy care we received in childhood and adolescence and demonstrate in the gentle, caring way that we respond to children. The Good Parent always has a caring attitude and positive view of the Child modes and can understand the origin and survival function of the Maladaptive Coping modes. The Good Parent is often a function that our clients have and use when dealing with others, particularly children, but do not apply to themselves. This may also be true for psychotherapists. We may be much kinder toward others than toward ourselves. Developing your own Good Parent is an important component of good self-care skills. Identifying the presence of a Good Parent toward others is an interim step toward being able to use it for oneself.

Getting to Know Your Healthy Adult Mode

 EXAMPLE: Ian's Healthy Adult Mode

Write about your Healthy Adult, as he or she exists today. For example, what strengths are you aware of?

I can be patient, reliable, kind, a good friend, loyal. I am reasonably intelligent and have completed an advanced degree. I can be open and loving. I am a good athlete and physically fit. I work hard. I know how to play also.

What percentage of a typical day are you in the Healthy Adult mode (0–100%)?

If I average the week, probably 85%. My issue is that I could be 100% for 4 days, then about 30%, and then back to 80 or 90%. So I appear inconsistent. When a Coping mode takes over, my Healthy Adult is gone.

How do you access your Healthy Adult?

I take a few deep breaths into my center, count to 3, and use soothing self-talk like "Calm down, Ian, no one is threatening you." Sometimes I use the Physical Grounding exercises from Module 1.

Write about the **Good Parent** part of your Healthy Adult mode.

This part of me is not well developed. My mother was not very affectionate, and my father, not at all. I am kind and loving toward my nephews, so I have some skills. I do find at times that my Demanding Critic pops out when they make mistakes or break things.

How do you access your Good Parent when a Child mode needs you?

I try to ask myself, "What would a good parent do?" I learned that question in an ST workshop and use it for clients when they are in Child modes.

EXERCISE. My Healthy Adult Mode

Now complete the form about your Healthy Adult mode.

Write about your Healthy Adult, as he or she exists today. For example, what strengths are you aware of?

What percentage of a typical day are you in the Healthy Adult mode (0–100%)?

How do you access your Healthy Adult?

Write about the **Good Parent** part of your Healthy Adult mode.

How do you access your Good Parent when a Child mode needs you?

Accessing Your Healthy Adult Mode via Messages

Table 2.8 provides examples of schema therapist interventions to meet various needs. In SP/SR you take on the limited reparenting functions of the therapist. One of the ways to do this is to develop messages to meet your present need, like a good parent would, and then access your Healthy Adult mode to provide the needed message. For the Coping and Critic modes you may want to speak from your Healthy Adult. For the Child modes, it may be more helpful to speak from the nurturing Good Parent part of your Healthy Adult mode. This idea of there being a part of the Healthy Adult mode that can care for you when Child modes are triggered is discussed further in Chapter 2.

EXAMPLE: Penny's Messages from Her Healthy Adult Mode

Following are some examples from Penny.

Mode	Healthy Adult Mode message
Maladaptive Coping mode *Detached Protector*	*It is OK for her to feel a little bit anxious—it won't kill her. Just take some breaths and don't make her detach.*
Dysfunctional Critic mode *Demanding Critic*	*She is doing well for a beginner. Stop criticizing and leave her alone!*
Messages from the Good Parent part of my Healthy Adult for my Child modes:	
Vulnerable Child mode	*I am here; I will support you and not let anything bad happen.*
Angry/Impulsive Child mode	*Not involved*
Happy Child mode	*Not involved*

 EXERCISE. Messages from My Healthy Adult Mode

Now develop some of your own messages. It may help to just ask yourself, "What would a good parent say or do?"

Mode	Healthy Adult Mode message
Maladaptive Coping mode	
Dysfunctional Critic mode	
Messages from the Good Parent part of my Healthy Adult for my Child modes:	
Vulnerable Child mode	
Angry/Impulsive Child mode	
Happy Child mode	

Using an ST Flashcard

In this exercise, you will organize the information you have collected into flashcard form. The ST flashcard acknowledges and validates the emotions involved and identifies its historical origin, the need involved, the survival coping behavior that is triggered, a reality check, and the action that would meet the need.

 EXAMPLE: Ian's ST Flashcard

The first example, from Ian (beginning below), goes through all of these steps. It is followed by a short version for ease of use.

IAN'S ST FLASHCARD

Right now I feel _anxious_ **because my** _Vulnerable Child_ **mode was triggered when** _I made a mistake with a client that was pointed out in supervision._

However, I know that this is probably my _Mistrust Abuse_ **schema being activated, Which I learned through** _my very critical father, who punished me severely for any mistake._

This schema(s) leads me to distort the degree to which _I am in danger of being vulnerable to humiliation._

So, even though I believe that _I will be put down and humiliated,_

The reality is that _I am an adult, my supervisor is not like my father, I am here to learn, so it is normal to make some mistakes._

Evidence supporting my Healthy Adult view includes: _My supervisor has never made fun of me for a mistake. She even has the statement "Make mistakes, that is how you learn" written on the chalkboard in the supervision room._

So, even though I feel like _going on the defensive to not feel vulnerable,_

I choose to do this instead: _Acknowledge that I missed my client's Detached Protector mode for most of the session and listen to feedback about how to improve._

Short Form

My Flashcard for <u>Mistrust–Abuse</u> (schema)

Even though I feel <u>terrified</u>

Mode Awareness: I know my reaction is based on my childhood experience of <u>no safety</u> and that my <u>mistrust-abuse</u> schema has been activated.

Mode Management: Although tempted to use my old coping mode, I will connect with my Healthy Adult mode and <u>ask my wife for validation,</u> as that will get my need met.

EXERCISE. My ST Flashcard

Now complete the long and short versions of the flashcards beginning below to help access your Healthy Adult mode. Complete the short flashcard form for ease of use and keep it in a place where you will frequently see it.

MY ST FLASHCARD

Right now I feel _____ because my _____ mode was triggered when _____

However, I know that this is probably my _____ schema being activated, Which I learned through _____

This schema(s) leads me to distort the degree to which _____

So, even though I believe that _____
The reality is that _____

Evidence supporting my Healthy Adult view includes: _____

So, even though I feel like _____
I choose to do this instead: _____

Short Form

My Flashcard for _____ **(schema)**
Even though I feel _____
Mode Awareness: I know my reaction is based on my childhood experience of _____
and that my _____ **schema has been activated.**
Mode Management: Although tempted to use my old coping mode, I will connect with my Healthy Adult mode and _____ **as that will get my need met.**

Self-Reflective Questions

How easy or difficult was it to describe your Healthy Adult mode? How did this exercise compare with describing your Dysfunctional modes? Was there any difference in how you felt while describing each?

_____

_____

_____

_____

_____

_____

_____

_____

_____

_____

_____

_____

_____

Comment on the process of using your awareness of modes to make choices that better meet your needs. Describe any difficulties. Was the process helpful? Unhelpful? At a cognitive level? At an emotional level?

_____

_____

_____

_____

_____

_____

_____

_____

_____

_____

_____

_____

_____

How do you access your Healthy Adult mode? Was the flashcard exercise helpful in connecting you to your Healthy Adult? Does anything interfere with this connection (e.g., the Critic mode)?

_____

_____

_____

_____

_____

_____

_____

_____

_____

_____

_____

_____

_____

_____

Have you noticed any changes in your thinking from doing the Cognitive Antidote work? What might you need to build into your personal or professional life to help you maintain your Healthy Adult mode connection? What situations might most challenge this connection?

_____

_____

_____

_____

_____

_____

_____

_____

_____

_____

_____

_____

_____

Are there any ways in which doing the mode model (including strengths) has changed the way you view yourself or the problem on which you chose to focus? If so, how?

_____

_____

_____

_____

_____

_____

_____

_____

_____

_____

_____

_____

_____

MODULE 13

Reviewing Progress
and Planning Further Change

Having the experience of identifying my underlying schemas, their activation,
and the triggering of various modes as a client is extremely helpful in being
able to understand and connect with my clients around this experience.
                                                                —SP/SR participant

In Module 13 we evaluate the effects of the work completed and repeat the Mode–
Schema Pie Chart assessment. We also determine whether moving on to experiential
mode work and healing for the Vulnerable Child mode is advisable at this time, and if
you do continue, what your goals would be.

Your Mode–Schema Pie Chart Review

It is time to do a second Mode–Schema Pie Chart. We suggest that you do the new
Mode–Schema Pie Chart **without referring back to the original one.**

 EXAMPLE: Julia's Mode–Schema Pie Chart #2

Julia's second Mode–Schema Pie Chart is shown on page 206.

JULIA'S MODE–SCHEMA CHART #2

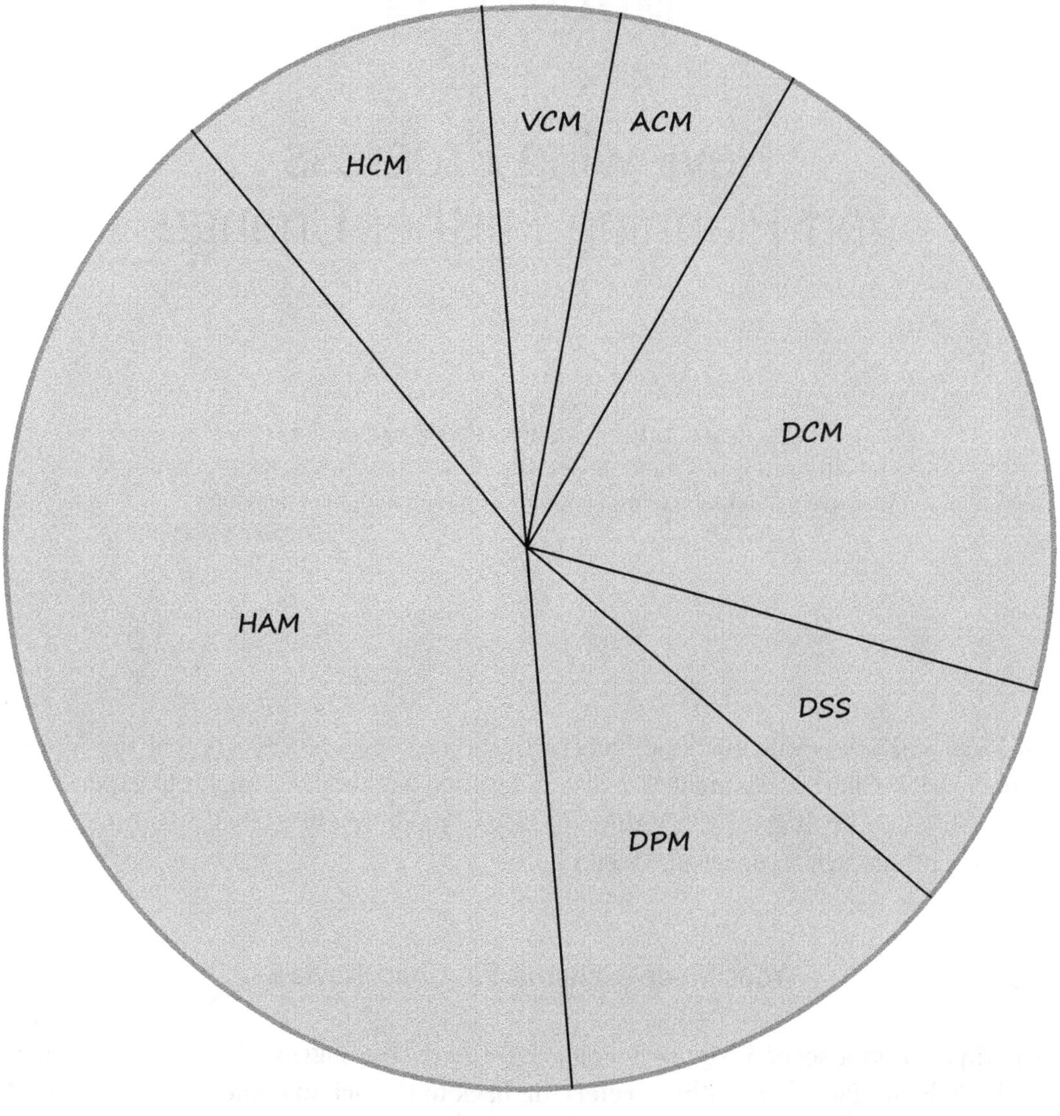

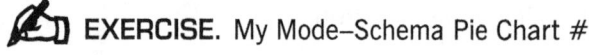

Mode labels key: VCM, Vulnerable Child; ACM, Angry Child; DPM, Detached Protector; DSS, Detached Self-Soother; DCM, Demanding Critic; HAM, Healthy Adult; HCM, Happy Child.

EXERCISE. My Mode–Schema Pie Chart #2

Now fill in your Mode–Schema Pie Chart on page 207.

MY MODE–SCHEMA CHART #2

Date: _____

Divide the circle with lines based on your experience of the modes over the last 2 weeks.

Mode labels key: VCM, Vulnerable Child; ACM, Angry Child; I/UCM, Angry/Undisciplined Child; DCM, Demanding Critic; PCM, Punitive Critic; AVM, Avoidant Coping; DPM, Detached Protector; DSS, Detached Self-Soother; OCM, Overcompensating; POC, Perfectionistic Overcontroller; BAM, Bully–Attack; SAM, Self-Aggrandizer; AAP, Attention/Approval Seeking; CSM, Compliant Surrenderer; PCM, Punitive Critic; DECM, Demanding Critic; HAM, Healthy Adult; HCM, Happy Child.

Look at your Mode–Schema Pie Chart. Has there been positive or negative change? Positive change would be decreases in the amount of time spent in the Maladaptive Coping modes or in the Dysfunctional Critic modes and increases in time spent in the Healthy Adult mode and Happy Child mode. Changes in the Innate Child modes are less clear. Sometimes people find that in the early sessions of ST, they become more aware of painful emotions and their Innate Child modes. Since this response may reflect increased awareness, we see a temporary increase in the Vulnerable Child mode as a positive change. However, this increased awareness may be temporarily uncomfortable. We liken it to recovering from frostbite. If your limbs hurt, it is a sign that they are healing and will return to normal function. If they remain numb, you are in trouble. Emotional healing may be painful, but it does lead to increased emotional health. In a similar way, a temporary increase in the Angry Child mode can be a positive change if a person was previously cut off from his or her anger. Generally, an increase in the time spent in the Impulsive or Undisciplined Child mode, however, is not usually a positive change.

 EXERCISE. Reviewing Your SP/SR Work

To make the decision whether to go further in self-practice utilizing additional experiential work on the Child modes and the Critic, answer the following questions.

---

1. How has your professional life been affected by your SP/SR work? For example supervision, client sessions, relationships with colleagues?

2. How has your personal life been affected?

---

3. Are you aware of any increased anxiety or depression?

4. Do you feel that you that you are benefiting from your SP/SR work and want to continue it at this time?

📌 *Notes.* Based upon your answers and overall experience of the first 12 modules of SP/SR, you can decide whether this is the time to go on to Part III of the program, repeat Part II, or stop the SP/SR work for now. It is also a time to evaluate whether you need the added support of a supervisor or personal therapist. This sort of review and evaluation is typical of ST: Decisions are made based upon a client's maladaptive modes, needs, and the strengths of his or her Healthy Adult mode, rather than on an arbitrary number of sessions. It is important when doing this kind of deeper-level or foundation work to go at the pace that fits for the client, who must continue to live his or her life while the therapy continues. Of course, this perspective also applies to your self-practice work.

The experiential work of Modules 14–18 is a critical component of ST. Without this component, you do not really "have" ST. As experienced schema therapists (we each have 25 years of working with this approach), we do not anticipate that the experiential work will be harmful or excessively upsetting for you. As discussed in the Practical Issues section of Chapter 3, experiential exercises are designed to be emotionally activating to varying degrees, which is why it is important to develop an effective safety plan. If you are under considerable stress, have experienced a significant trauma or loss, or are in a period of grief, you may want to delay going further with the ST SP/SR program.

You may want to look at the experiential work in Modules 14–18 to see if this is the time for you to do Vulnerable Child mode work. Keep in mind that we ask our clients to do this work in ST, albeit with the support of a therapist. It is possible to skip any of the modules and go on to Modules 19 and 20, which focus on strengthening the healthy modes—Happy Child and Healthy Adult—and then complete the summary self-reflection. However, we do encourage you to try Modules 14–18 for a number of reasons. As discussed in Chapter 3, ST requires therapists to be authentically present in sessions. In turn, this presence requires a good deal of self-awareness and comfort with strong emotions. We ask our patients to do the exercises in Modules 14–18. If a therapist is not able to take a look at his or her Vulnerable Child mode experience and emotional needs, ST may not be the right model for that therapist to use.

Self-Practice Review of Change Accomplished by Mode

To help decide about continuing SP/SR work, we suggest that you review the positive change that you have accomplished in each mode and what additional work may be needed. Penny's self-practice review is shown beginning below.

 PENNY'S SELF-PRACTICE REVIEW

Schemas	Unrelenting Standards I have also become aware that Defectiveness/Shame is a related schema that may trigger my Overcompensating mode.
Maladaptive Coping mode	Perfectionistic Overcontroller
What has changed?	I am aware of when this mode is triggered with others, so I can tone it down some. I know that when my voice starts to sound like my mother's, I need to take a few breaths and stop the escalation.
What work is still left to do?	The mode is triggered a lot still. I need to notice it more when it takes over and drives me to excess work.
Dysfunctional Critic mode	Demanding Critic
What has changed?	Again, I am aware of this mode being triggered. I use my Good Parent message to neutralize the Critic.
What work is still left to do?	I still feel the criticism and driving of my Critic a good deal. I would like to do something about the effects of the Critic on my Vulnerable Child.

Vulnerable Child mode	Sad and lonely child
What has changed?	I am aware of Little Penny's needs at times when I am working excessive hours. She would like to have time to play.
What work is still left to do?	I need to pay attention to the need to play or relax and devote some time just to that.
Other Child mode (specify type)	Undisciplined Child
What has changed?	I see the times when I just won't do more work as my way to balance work and play.
What work is still left to do?	It would be more effective if I allowed time to play rather than working relentlessly and then rebelling and doing nothing. When that happens, I cannot completely enjoy the break, as my Critic gets active.
Happy Child mode	
What has changed?	Not much.
What work is still left to do?	I need to explore this aspect of myself more.
Healthy Adult mode	
What has changed?	I am more aware of accessing this part of myself rather than going with dysfunctional modes that are triggered.
What work is still left to do?	I have made progress with the Perfectionistic Overcontroller and my Critic, but I still cut off frequently when I start noticing the sadness or loneliness of my Little Penny. She has missed a lot due to my excessive working and ignoring her.

 EXERCISE. My Self-Practice Review

Complete your self-practice review on pages 212–213.

MY SELF-PRACTICE REVIEW

Schemas	
Maladaptive Coping mode	
What has changed?	
What work is still left to do?	
Dysfunctional Critic mode	
What has changed?	
What work is still left to do?	
Vulnerable Child mode	
What has changed?	
What work is still left to do?	
Other Child mode (specify type)	
What has changed?	
What work is still left to do?	

Happy Child mode	
What has changed?	
What work is still left to do?	
Healthy Adult mode	
What has changed?	
What work is still left to do?	

From *Experiencing Schema Therapy from the Inside Out: A Self-Practice/Self-Reflection Workbook for Therapists* by Joan M. Farrell and Ida A. Shaw. Copyright © 2018 The Guilford Press. Permission to photocopy this form is granted to purchasers of this book for personal use only (see copyright page for details). Purchasers can download additional copies of this form (see the box at the end of the table of contents).

If you are going to continue SP/SR work, it is time to update your goals by mode to reflect the work you have done and your increased understanding of your identified problem.

 EXAMPLE: Penny's Goals by Mode for Continuing SP/SR Work

Vulnerable Child mode Little Penny	Increase my awareness of Little Penny—her feelings and needs.
Other Child mode Little Rebel	Use the presence of this mode as a signal that I need some time off to play or relax.
Maladaptive Coping mode Miss Perfection	Increase my awareness of times when I am micro-managing students and let it go.
Dysfunctional Critic mode The Slave Driver	Shout her out when she criticizes taking time off. She is not in charge.
Healthy Adult mode Good Parent Penny	Be able to listen to Little Penny and commit to meeting her needs.
Happy Child mode Happy Child Penny	I need to learn to play and let myself fully enjoy it.

EXERCISE. My Goals by Mode for Continuing SP/SR Work

Describe your goals by mode for continuing SP/SR work below.

Vulnerable Child mode	
Other Child mode	
Maladaptive Coping mode	
Dysfunctional Critic mode	
Healthy Adult mode	
Happy Child mode	

A Pros and Cons List for Continuing SP/SR Work

To make this decision, it is useful to develop a Pros and Cons List with the information you gathered in the last two exercises.

EXAMPLE: Ian's Pros and Cons List for Continuing SP/SR Work

Ian's Pros and Cons List appears beginning below. Ian decided to continue SP/SR work, as the benefits appeared to outweigh the costs. He also realized that there were some schema messages in the Cons column—for example, the message of entitlement.

IAN'S PROS AND CONS LIST FOR CONTINUING SP/SR WORK

Reasons to continue SP/SR work	Reasons to stop SP/SR work
1. I still have some work to do with reducing the number of times my Bully–Attack mode takes over at work and at home. 2. I feel shame or embarrassment less when I access my Healthy Ian rather than Bully Ian. 3. I need the feedback my supervisor gives to increase my ST skills.	• I've changed enough; this is hard work • Why can't they just understand that I am sensitive to criticism and lay off? Why do I have to change? • I am good the way I am. • It takes time away from playing sports, which I love.

4. I am responsible for my behavior; no one else is.
5. I want to have a closer, more secure relationship with my wife—I don't want to hurt her and push her away.
6. I don't want to be seen as a "hothead" at work—it doesn't look good for a psychotherapist.
7. I still get time for sports.

EXERCISE. My Pros and Cons List for Continuing SP/SR Work

Using all the information that you have gathered regarding your experience of SP/SR, develop a Pros and Cons List to decide whether to continue.

PROS AND CONS LIST FOR CONTINUING SP/SR WORK

Reasons to continue SP/SR work	Reasons to stop SP/SR work

What is your decision?

Self-Reflective Questions

You have now completed more than half of the workbook. How would you summarize your overall reaction to the self-practice exercises so far?

_____

_____

_____

_____

_____

_____

_____

_____

_____

_____

_____

_____

What have you discovered about yourself in this process? Is your discovery more in the "personal" or "therapist" self? Have any of your experiences of self-practice particularly stood out for you?

_____

_____

_____

_____

_____

_____

_____

_____

_____

_____

_____

_____

_____

_____

How would you summarize your overall reaction to the self-reflective questions so far? Can you identify any difficulties with the reflective process? Are there any steps you can take to improve this experience for yourself?

_____

_____

_____

_____

_____

_____

_____

_____

_____

_____

_____

_____

_____

What was your experience of reviewing your progress like for you? How difficult was it? Were you surprised by any of the results? Did you notice any self-criticism relating to your engagement with SP/SR? If so, which mode is involved?

_____

_____

_____

_____

_____

_____

_____

_____

_____

_____

_____

_____

Does completing this evaluation of progress in self-practice give you any additional insight into how a client feels when doing the same thing? Will you change the way you conduct reviews with clients based upon your experience?

_____

_____

_____

_____

_____

_____

_____

_____

_____

_____

_____

_____

_____

Can you bring to mind a particular client who may be experiencing difficulty in progressing? Is there anything that you have learned from reviewing your own progress that might be relevant for this client? If so, how will you put this new understanding into practice? When? Where? How?

_____

_____

_____

_____

_____

_____

_____

_____

_____

_____

_____

_____

_____

PART V

Experiential Mode Change Work

If you have decided to continue with your SP/SR work in Part V of the workbook, you will find experiential, emotion-focused interventions for the Innate Child modes and the interference of the Dysfunctional Critic modes. These interventions operate at the level of emotion and provide the corrective emotional experiences necessary to change schemas. Young (Young et al., 2003) describes this component of ST as fighting schemas on the affective level. Learning occurs more dramatically and faster in the presence of affect. Experiential interventions evoke affect. The main experiential interventions of ST are imagery work, including imagery rescripting, mode dialogues, the use of transitional objects, play, and other creative and symbolizing work (e.g., Critic effigies, beads on a bracelet to represent Healthy Adult mode strengths). Some interventions target early developmental levels and facilitate internalizing the therapist as a "Good Parent" and learning to self-soothe. Many corrective emotional experiences like these can be facilitated in ST and ST self-practice. These are the interventions ST adds to CBT that can change the felt aspect of schemas and modes. Patients often tell us, "I know in my head that I am not worthless, but I *feel* bad and worthless." The experiential interventions of Modules 14 through 18 address the latter aspect of experience.

Module 14 begins this section by addressing the Angry or Impulsive/Undisciplined Child mode. It is the Angry Child mode that expresses the child's feelings about having a core need go unmet. At the most basic level it is an infant crying or screaming when hungry, wet, cold, etc. The Vulnerable Child mode contains the discomfort of the unmet need and underlies the Angry Child mode. In **Module 15** we focus on awareness of the Vulnerable Child and building self-compassion. This is followed in **Module 16** by a Mode Management Plan to get unmet needs met by accessing the "Good Parent" skills of your Healthy Adult mode. The Dysfunctional Critic modes can interfere with a person's efforts to take action to meet his or her own needs. **Module 17** describes experiential interventions to diminish the Critic's power. The last module of this section, **Module 18,** presents some introductory imagery rescripting to help heal the Vulnerable Child mode. Experiences that are appropriate to rescript in self-practice are described.

Awareness of Your Angry or Impulsive/Undisciplined Child Mode

> Because I had had the experience of being surprised at the depth of my own anger when I experienced release after pulling the towel to try to unseat my partner exercise, I can tell a client with authority that using a physical intervention to release anger he or she is not entirely aware of can lead to some important information. I don't feel that it is silly any more.
>
> —SP/SR participant

In Module 14 you will work with your Angry and/or Impulsive/Undisciplined Child mode by developing a Mode Management Plan and an ST flashcard.

Notes. Anger is the primary feeling of the Angry Child mode. When you are in this mode, you may feel angry, enraged, frustrated, or annoyed, and you may vent your anger in a manner that is not seen as appropriate for an adult or that is "too big" for the immediate situation. Your expression may be similar to the tantrum of a child with an unmet need such as hunger, protection, or comfort. Your response may go beyond the expression of anger to impulsive action. When action is taken to meet the underlying need, the Impulsive Child mode has been triggered. When you are in the Impulsive Child mode, you may take action without any thought to possible negative consequences. In the Impulsive Child mode you may feel what the Angry Child feels, but also act in a selfish or uncontrolled manner to get your needs met, and you may appear "spoiled." You may even act very impulsively without being aware of any anger. If this is the case, we call it the Impulsive Child mode rather than Angry Child mode. Another variant of this mode is called the Undisciplined Child mode. In this mode, disciplined action is not taken; for example, instead of finishing an assessment report due the next day, you watch reality TV shows. It is a form of meeting a noncore need without considering your long-term goals, like keeping your job.

These three modes—Angry, Impulsive, and Undisciplined—are innate reactions to childhood needs not being met. They are triggered in adult life when a situation activates an EMS. Thus, the reaction is not just to the immediate situation, but also to childhood situations where needs were not met. When one is in the Healthy Adult mode, anger is an emotion that is felt and expressed in an assertive manner that matches the intensity and need of the situation. When anger is expressed in a manner disproportionate to the present situation, such as using verbal aggression, name-calling, yelling, or physical aggression, it is a clue that a dysfunctional mode is involved. The problem with the expressions of these modes is twofold: They usually do not get the underlying need met, and they have negative consequences in terms of how you are viewed by others and on interpersonal relationships.

Many people with psychological problems have never had a healthy adult model to show them how a child who is angry should be responded to and helped to safely express the anger. Often they were either punished for the expression of anger or given the message that it is "not OK" to be angry. So they never learned how to deal with the needs of their Angry Child mode. Some people have suppressed their Angry Child mode for such a long time that it takes a while for them to even discover their angry feelings. Others are afraid of their anger and think that they have no control when in Angry Child mode. They often learn growing up that anger is a "bad" thing—it means someone will be yelled at, hit, punished severely. Their only models of anger may have been scary adults who are out of control. They fear that they will lose control or "go crazy" if they allow any anger to be present. For these clients, including those with personality disorders, those who have experienced physical abuse, and those who have less access to their Healthy Adult Mode, setting up safe venting can be more difficult. This can be worked on slowly in therapist-led sessions in a number of ways that provide adequate safety and even a fun element (see Farrell & Shaw, 2012; Farrell, Reiss, & Shaw, 2014).

It is important that when you or your clients are in the Angry Child mode, you have a safe way to express your anger, verbalize what makes you angry, and express your need. Usually it is not just one thing but many and even a large backlog. From your Healthy Adult mode it is important to listen to the Angry Child mode, hear the underlying need, take it seriously, and remember all of it. In doing so, you provide self-validation that the anger is understandable based upon childhood experiences. After venting and validation, it is important to look at what the needs of the Angry Child are and what the options are for getting them filled. It is also important to look at how he or she can deal with anger in the future to be able to express it effectively and safely—without damaging self, others, or your relationships.

Awareness of Your Angry or Impulsive/Undisciplined Child Mode

In self-practice, we assume some amount of Healthy Adult mode in therapists and therefore provide a relatively mild intervention to deal with the Angry Child mode. If this mode is one of particular difficulty for you, you may want to take this work into self-therapy with a schema therapist. In Module 14, choose the mode that affects your identified problem from the Angry Child or Impulsive/Undisciplined Child mode.

 EXAMPLE: Ian's Angry Child Mode Experience

> I have been trying to share household tasks more evenly with my wife. Consequently, I am taking on some tasks that are new for me, like dealing with recyclables. I tend to wait until the last minute before they are being picked up, so I get all of them for the week. This makes my wife think that I am not going to remember to prepare them for pickup. When she asked me for the second time whether I was going to get them ready, I blew up, ranting and raving and telling her that she could "damn well do it yourself if you were going to nag me." This led to my wife's withdrawing in tears, and after a bit of time had passed, I felt like a "monster." As I reflected on my behavior, I realized that my Defectiveness schema had been activated, which triggered my Angry Child mode. I realized that I reacted so intensely due to childhood experiences with my perfectionistic and belittling father. I felt shame for talking to my wife as I had and embarrassed for making such a big deal of it. It was way too small a thing to explain the intensity of my reaction.

 EXAMPLE: Ian's Analysis of His Angry Child Mode Awareness

Clues that a Child mode reaction is triggered

I felt intense anger, started yelling right away, and said things to my wife that I don't usually feel or believe. It was way too big a response to her asking a question.

What need is involved?

Validation as competent and reliable, autonomy, respect

What EMS has been activated?

Defectiveness/Shame

What memory is involved?

My dad yelling at me for every little thing he thought I did wrong—forgetting to take out the garbage, saying I was useless and lazy.

What action do I usually take?

I start yelling immediately at the person before I even think. I call him or her names.

What is the usual result? Is my need met?

With my wife, she cries and goes away. I feel guilty and bad. With colleagues, they try to set limits, then walk off disgusted. I am finding out that few colleagues will work with me now.

EXAMPLE: Julia's Undisciplined Child Experience

> My Child mode is the Undisciplined type. At times when I have a boring task to do in the evening when I get home from work, I can easily be lured away by a TV show or deciding to call a friend and chat for hours. Then I realize that I am really tied, and it is midnight, and I haven't gotten anything done.

Here is what Julia's Mode Awareness Summary looks like.

 EXAMPLE: Julia's Analysis of Her Undisciplined Child Mode Awareness

---

Clues that a Child mode reaction is triggered

I feel restless and just don't want to go over the case notes I need to review for supervision tomorrow. I am bored and just can't seem to get down to work.

What need is involved?

Self-control

What EMS has been activated?

Insufficient self-control, self-discipline

What memory is involved?

Having to write out Latin case endings endless times until I could recite them on under a minute. I was so bored.

What action do I usually take?

I blow it off and begin to watch a series on cable. That is what I want to do.

What is the usual result? Is my need met?

I am not prepared the next day and feel incompetent. My supervisor says she is disappointed with my analysis—that it sounds like a put little time in.

No, I didn't use any self-control.

 EXERCISE. My Analysis of My Angry or Impulsive/Undisciplined Child Mode

Now complete the same form to analyze your awareness of the Child mode related to your identified problem.

MY ANALYSIS OF MY ANGRY OR IMPULSIVE/UNDISCIPLINED CHILD MODE

Clues that a Child mode reaction is triggered

What need is involved?

What EMS has been activated?

What memory is involved?

What action do I usually take?

What is the usual result?

Is my need met?

Your Mode Management Plan

Awareness is the first step in mode change. The next is making a plan for how you will respond in a healthier way—one that will better meet your needs—when a mode is triggered.

 EXAMPLES: Ian's and Julia's Mode Management Plans

Based upon their awareness analysis above, Ian and Julia completed Mode Management Plans on pages 228–229.

IAN'S ANGRY CHILD MODE MANAGEMENT PLAN

What situations does this mode get triggered in?	When I feel criticized or told what to do.
Which EMS triggers this mode?	Defectiveness/Shame
What need is involved?	Validation, autonomy
How can I use my awareness of the this mode to stop and make a choice?	I can work to recognize clues that my Angry Child mode is being triggered before I have an outburst. I can notice the feeling of heat moving up my neck to my face and be aware of the thought "Don't tell me what to do."
How could I vent the surplus anger safely, if needed? Try it.	I can take three deep breaths whenever I became aware of either clue, and if I still feel intense anger, I can take a time-out and ask to discuss the issue later.
How could I get the need met in a healthy way? Try it.	I can tell Sarah why I react so strongly to reminders. I can take some action to get my need to be treated as someone competent and worthy met by explaining to Sarah that I have a reminder to deal with the recyclables that will pop up on my computer 30 minutes before pickup. I can tell her it is upsetting to be repeatedly reminded and ask her to please not remind me, but to let me do it myself.
What was the result and was my need met?	She said she understood my feelings based on my history and that she knew I was competent and responsible. She agreed to let me use my plan to remember time limits for chores. Yes.
What message from my Healthy Adult can I use as an "antidote" for this mode?	"I understand why you feel so angry and humiliated because of the way Dad treated you, but this is not Dad, it is Sarah, and she is not trying to put you down or criticize you."

JULIA'S UNDISCIPLINED CHILD MODE MANAGEMENT PLAN

What situations does this mode get triggered in?	When I am on a deadline and need to get down to work.
Which EMS triggers this mode?	Insufficient self-control or self-discipline
What need is involved?	Self-control

How can I use my awareness of the this mode to stop and make a choice?	When I sit down and start to roam through the cable channels, I need to stop and get to the work I need to do.
How could I vent the surplus anger safely, if needed? Try it.	I could just complain out loud about the need to work instead of being free to play.
How could I get the need met in a healthy way? Try it.	I could make sure that I have some time to relax and have entertainment in the evening, but also allot adequate time to get my work done.
What was the result and was my need met?	I felt much better the next day when I was prepared for supervision, and I felt satisfied that I could also watch one installment of the series.
What message from my Healthy Adult can I use as an "antidote" for this mode?	"We have to spend some time in the evening preparing for the next day's work, but we will also have some time for fun. Work first, then we are free to play."

Notes. As you can see in Ian's example, the disruption of the Angry/Impulsive Child mode can be a relatively simple problem to resolve as an adult in the present, but could damage a relationship if it was not understood, discussed, and a management plan formed. A goal of ST is that your Healthy Adult mode is able to help your Angry Child mode vent his or her anger in a nondamaging way and, over time, channel that anger into healthy assertive skills. You can use these skills from your Healthy Adult mode to clarify your personal boundaries, express your needs, and reach your goals. In the same way, for Julia's example, her awareness that she was making a choice to allow her Undisciplined Child mode to take over allowed her to consider the consequences and face finding a way to manage her need for play with the need for self-control.

The Mode Management Plan employs cognitive, experiential, and behavioral pattern-breaking interventions. In Ian's example, the **cognitive level** is addressed via reality testing: *Sarah is not Dad, she is not trying to belittle me.* The **experiential level** is addressed by the validation from Sarah: *She said she understood my feelings and knew that I was competent and responsible. It felt good to hear that.* The **behavioral pattern-breaking component** is also present: *I will notice my Angry Child mode being triggered and take action to delay until I can access my Healthy Adult mode.*

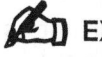 **EXERCISE.** My Mode Management Plan for the Angry or Impulsive/Undisciplined Child Mode

Now make a Mode Management Plan for your Angry/Impulsive Child mode.

MY ANGRY OR IMPULSIVE/UNDISCIPLINED CHILD MODE
MANAGEMENT PLAN

What situations does this mode get triggered in?	
Which EMS triggers this mode?	
What need is involved?	
How can I use my awareness of the this mode to stop and make a choice?	
How could I vent the surplus anger safely, if needed? Try it.	
How could I get the need met in a healthy way? Try it.	
What was the result and was my need met?	
What message from my Healthy Adult can I use as an "antidote" for this mode?	

An ST Antidote Flashcard

Next, we summarize each Mode Management Plan in a shortened form as a flashcard to keep visible to support behavioral pattern breaking. Flashcards are important as reminders of the awareness about maladaptive modes that has been gained, and they provide an alternate plan in a "fight, flight, or freeze" situation: the choice to access the Healthy Adult mode.

EXAMPLE: Ian's Angry Child Flashcard and Julia's Undisciplined Child Flashcard

> **Ian:** When I notice that my anger feels bigger than the present, I will access my Healthy Ian part, take three deep breaths, and identify what I need and how I can get it in an adult way. I will tell Angry Ian that I understand his intense feelings based on how dad treated me.

> **Julia:** When I get home after work and feel the pull to the recliner in the TV room, I will access Healthy Adult Julia and decide the amount of time I need for work and how much time I have to play. Since I know how strong Undisciplined Julia can be, I will make sure that the plan is to do the needed work for tomorrow first, then allow myself the TV reward.

EXERCISE. My Angry or Impulsive/Undisciplined Child Mode Flashcard

>

ASSIGNMENT

Use your Mode Management Plan and flashcard until you move on to the next module. Record the results and your experience with it here.

>

Self-Reflective Questions

What was your overall immediate reaction to doing the self-practice exercises for the Angry or Impulsive/Undisciplined Child mode? Was it easy, difficult, or uncomfortable thinking about this part of yourself? Did you experience any particular emotions, bodily sensations, or thoughts while you were doing the exercises?

_____

_____

_____

_____

_____

_____

_____

_____

_____

_____

_____

What are your childhood memories of being in one of these Child modes? How were you responded to? Was your underlying need understood or met?

_____

_____

_____

_____

_____

_____

_____

_____

_____

_____

_____

_____

When you have experienced one of these Child modes, do you ever flip to another mode? If so, which one?

_____

_____

_____

_____

_____

_____

_____

_____

_____

_____

_____

_____

_____

What is the attitude of your internal Good Parent to your Angry or Impulsive/Undisciplined Child?

_____

_____

_____

_____

_____

_____

_____

_____

_____

_____

_____

_____

After your experience of these mode exercises from the inside out, do you have any different understanding of your clients' experiences of these modes? Is there anything you will do differently in your work with these modes with your clients?

_____

_____

_____

_____

_____

_____

_____

_____

_____

_____

_____

_____

MODULE 15

Awareness of
Your Vulnerable Child Mode

I think that a therapist must be able to reach his or her own vulnerable
child and look at it, so as not to be overwhelmed by it—then you can
empathize with the vulnerable part of the client. I was surprised at how
much emotion I felt in the imagery exercise when I discovered that the
little lonely child was me. I can really see using this with my clients.
—SP/SR participant

Module 15 focuses on identifying the feelings and needs that are present when you
are in the Vulnerable Child mode. We use experiential interventions, including
imagery, to be able to access the feelings and needs that are present when you are in this
mode and to begin to meet the needs present in a healthy way.

Notes. In the Vulnerable Child mode we experience the core childhood needs that
were not fully met in our childhoods along with the feelings from those experiences.
These emotions of fear, anxiety, sadness, loneliness, abandonment, etc., are very strong
and can even feel as if they threaten our survival. In the Vulnerable Child mode we feel
like we are, once again, a helpless, needy child. In the ST model, the survival action
(fight, flight, or freeze) taken to deal with the need of the Vulnerable Child mode is
conceptualized as among the Maladaptive Coping modes. These modes were discussed
and worked with in Modules 8 and 9. The negative messages that reflect the core beliefs
of EMS and can trigger the Vulnerable Child mode are conceptualized as the Dysfunctional Critic mode. This mode is described and worked with using cognitive and behavioral interventions in Modules 10 and 11 and experiential interventions in Module 17.

For our clients, particularly those with personality disorders, many of the core needs
of childhood were not met in extreme ways. They may not have been safe, protected,
nurtured, or loved and may have been abandoned, abused, and/or neglected. For many
therapists, the failure of the early environment was not as extreme. It may have been

that validation was infrequent and unintentional: Perhaps parents were occupied with careers, one of the siblings was ill and required extra care, a childhood illness required long hospitalization and time away from parents; or possibly a parent was in the military or simply emotionally inhibited and had difficulty being physically affectionate, etc. Of course, a therapist's childhood environment may have been as extreme as any client's. Differences that lead to unmet childhood needs also occur as a result of the mismatch between a child's temperament and those of his or her parents. Lack of compatible temperaments and the failure to accurately assess and understand the needs of a temperamentally different child also play a role in the adequacy of the childhood environment. Needs may have been met in early childhood, but not in adolescence when needs related to autonomy and emotional expression are the focus. Here the role of teachers, coaches, and the peer group take on primary importance. The Vulnerable Child mode thus falls along a continuum from that of a very young toddler (who is nonverbal) to an adolescent. It is important to consider the age of the Vulnerable Child mode for clients and in working with your own Child modes.

Description of the Vulnerable Child mode	How the Vulnerable Child mode develops	Possible schemas involved
In this mode, you may feel sad, frantic, frightened, unloved, lost, and/or lonely. You may feel helpless and utterly alone and obsessed with finding someone who will take care of you. You may look to others to rescue you. An adult in this mode will feel like a young child, to varying degrees.	This mode develops when any of the core childhood needs is not met or is met sporadically or unpredictably. You may have been left alone for long periods; received inadequate comfort, safety, and nurturing; been punished harshly, physically or emotionally; love may have been withheld based upon performance or harsh criticism given. In essence, there was some inadequacy in your core needs being met.	Abandonment Mistrust–abuse Emotional deprivation, Defectiveness/Shame Social isolation/alienation Dependence/incompetence Vulnerability to harm or illness Enmeshment/undeveloped self Negativity/pessimism

Young (Young et al., 2003) describes a person in the Vulnerable Child mode as like a young child in the world who needs the care of adults in order to survive, but is not getting that care. The severity of the Vulnerable Child mode, like the age range to which it applies, can be viewed along a continuum in relation to how much Healthy Adult mode is present at the same time and able to observe and intervene. The more the Healthy Adult mode is present, the less severe is the Vulnerable Child's response. In this mode you may reject or be confused by the intensity of these feelings. You may also shut down the feelings of this mode before any memory or content develops or experience it as embarrassing or representing weakness. Early caretakers may have punished you for expressing your needs, or you may have taken away messages about feelings and needs being wrong from caretakers' lack of response. You may have been called "too needy" or you may have felt "too needy" when in this mode. It is helpful to keep in mind that these feelings come from the experience in childhood of your *normal needs* not being adequately met.

 EXAMPLE: Penny's Vulnerable Child Mode

> *Occasionally out of the blue, I feel myself tearing up. My immediate response is to jump into a cognitive-analytic stance, asking myself, "What is this about?" This move to analyze the feeling is usually enough for it to disappear (most likely into the Detached Protector mode). Thus I am not able to make use of the information that my tears may have given me.*

Because Penny quickly detaches from the physical sensations and feelings of her Vulnerable Child mode, she never finds out what content or memory is present along with a possibly unmet need.

Connecting with Your Vulnerable Child Mode

Can you get an image of yourself as a little child? People vary in how well they are able to see this kind of image or experience this connection with the Vulnerable Child part of them. Sometimes the images people see are re-creations of pictures they have of themselves as children at different ages. Pictures can also be used to facilitate a connection in imagery or just to activate feelings, thoughts, and memories.

 EXAMPLE: Julia's Way of Connecting with Her Vulnerable Child Mode

> *I remember a picture of me at my first birthday party. I was dressed up like a little doll in a frilly party dress, hair carefully curled. In the picture, I am in front of my birthday cake and have a dot of frosting carefully placed upon my nose. The picture was obviously staged. I am not smiling, but rather look a bit frightened. To me this picture represents the image of the perfect little girl my mother required, and I am able to connect strongly with that little girl.*

EXERCISE. Connecting with Your Vulnerable Child Mode

1. Find a picture of yourself as a child that you can connect with strongly. If you do not have such a picture, either draw one or take a picture from a magazine that resembles you as a child and represents the feelings that occur when you are in the Vulnerable Child mode. Describe the child in the picture here:

2. What do you think the child was feeling? What are you feeling right now?

3. What do you think the child was thinking? What are your thoughts now?

4. What did the child need? What do you need now?

5. Who was there to fill the need? How well was it filled? How is it filled when you experience it today?

6. How can you make a connection with this child?

Keep the picture of yourself as a child available as you are doing the work in Modules 16–18. If it is difficult for you to get a visual image, look at the picture instead. We use these same exercises to assist clients in accessing a Vulnerable Child mode image. Summarize your information about your experience of this mode in the following chart.

MY VULNERABLE CHILD MODE EXPERIENCE

Thoughts

Feelings

Physical sensations

Memories

Needs

EXERCISE. "The Lonely, Scared Little Child on the Street" Imagery Exercise

It is important to begin to develop some compassion for the little child you were and for yourself when this mode is present in your current life. A person in the Vulnerable Child mode needs a good parent to meet his or her needs. An important goal of ST is to develop acceptance and compassion for the Vulnerable Child mode part of you and to develop a "Good Parent" component of your Healthy Adult mode who can respond in the positive and caring way that you would with a beloved young child.

Notes. In ST we use this imagery exercise to assess the client's "Good Parent" skills, which include an acceptance of the idea that all children have core needs that deserve to be met. We also assess the client's relationship with his or Vulnerable Child mode. We follow this same process in the workbook. This exercise the first step in starting to find your inner Good Parent, which we see as the part of the Healthy Adult Mode that will eventually care for your needs when you are in the Vulnerable Child mode.

Imagery Exercise, Part I

There are two different ways for you to approach this exercise: You could read the instructions into a recorder and play them back, or read a section at a time and then follow that section's instructions. The recording method is closer to what the client experiences in a session.

Instructions: Close your eyes or look down and try to imagine the situation that we will describe to you. Just be aware of any thought, feeling, or mode that is present. Change the gender of the child to match your own.

> "You are walking down the street toward your home, and you see a small child ahead of you. Your first reaction is that she is too young to be out alone, only 3 or 4 years old. As you get closer to the little child, you notice that she is crying and her head is hanging down. When she sees you, she keeps her head down, but raises a hand up to you in an imploring way."

1. What do you do?

2. How do you feel?

3. What thoughts are you aware of?

4. How do you continue to try to take care of her? Describe the actions that you take.

Imagery Exercise, Part II

"So, once again you are leaving your home, and you see a little child sitting in the street crying. You walk up to the child, murmuring comforting things. This time as you get closer, the child raises both arms toward you to be picked up. You decide to pick the child up, and, as you do, you realize that it is *you* as a little child."

---

1. What do you do?

2. How do you feel?

3. What thoughts are you aware of?

4. How do you continue to try to take care of your little child? Describe the actions you take here and anything that interferes with your taking care of your little Vulnerable Child.

🖈 *Notes.* This exercise can be quite emotionally evocative. It is a first step in asking clients to care for themselves when they are in the Vulnerable Child mode. This exercise gives you information about how much or little compassion the client has for his or her Vulnerable Child mode. Doing the imagery yourself will give you feedback about your level of compassion for your Vulnerable Child mode. Many clients have an appropriate and effective response to the stranger-child, but a negative reaction when the child is identified as their Vulnerable Child. They express dislike for that child or say that they "don't know what to do with her." This is not due to a skills deficit but rather to a discrimination error in not matching caretaking skills they use with others to meet the needs of their own Vulnerable Child. Some therapists in self-practice say that the exercise is more difficult in some way when they are the child than when the child is a stranger. Other therapists enjoy the experience of caring for their own little Vulnerable Child. These responses provide openings with clients to introduce the idea of compassion for the little children they were, who had the same universal needs as the little lonely stranger-child in the imagery has. We remind our clients that all children deserve to have these universal needs met, and we ask pointed questions such as "How does a young innocent child become bad in your eyes?"

The occasional client says that he or she has no "Good Parent." We have those clients come into the image to watch exactly how we take care of the little child, so that they can begin to build their own Good Parents. We see a client's Good Parent as a representation of any good parenting he or she received throughout life, including from prior therapists, and what they are getting from us in the limited reparenting of ST. The Good Parent is a building block of the Healthy Adult mode. We have found that, most often, clients have Good Parent skills, but schemas or the Dysfunctional Critic modes prevent them using these skills for themselves. The interference of the Critic modes is further addressed in Module 18.

✍ EXERCISE. Repetition of the Imagery Exercise

Repeat Part II of the imagery exercise, this time with the knowledge that you will meet your own Vulnerable Child mode. In imagery, let your "little child" take in all of the care and warmth that you have to give. Take his or her little hand in yours and give him or her a caring message from you—for example: "I love you just the way you are"; "You are a wonderful, special little child, and I will protect you and always be there for you." If these messages feel difficult, you can always say, "I am learning that you deserved to be loved and cared for and to have your needs met." Write this message in the following box and on an index card and place it where you will see it often.

Self-Reflective Questions

What was your overall immediate reaction to doing the self-practice exercises? Was it easy, difficult, or uncomfortable thinking about yourself in this way? Did you experience any particular emotions, bodily sensations, or thoughts while you were doing the exercises?

_____

_____

_____

_____

_____

_____

_____

_____

_____

_____

_____

_____

_____

_____

How comfortable were you with the use of an imagery exercise? Can you see using it with your clients?

_____

_____

_____

_____

_____

_____

_____

_____

_____

_____

_____

_____

_____

_____

Were you surprised by anything in your reaction to your Vulnerable Child mode? Were any modes triggered? For example, did the Dysfunctional Critic tell your little Vulnerable Child mode to "Shape up, stop crying, etc"? Were any schemas activated—for example, Self-Sacrifice, Defectiveness/Shame, Unrelenting Standards, or others?

_____

_____

_____

_____

_____

_____

_____

_____

_____

_____

_____

_____

_____

_____

Were you surprised by anything in your reaction to the "The Lonely, Scared Little Child on the Street" exercise? Did you feel competent to identify and respond to that little child's needs?

_____

_____

_____

_____

_____

_____

_____

_____

_____

_____

_____

_____

_____

_____

Did you respond in the same way to the needs of your Vulnerable Child mode as to those of the stranger-child, or was your response different? Did you identify any barriers to self-compassion?

MODULE 16

A Management Plan
for Your Vulnerable Child Mode

> The Vulnerable Child work has helped me to be less self-critical and more compassionate toward myself. I understand my clients better during their process. I am not afraid of acknowledging my vulnerable side to clients, and I connect better when they feel vulnerable because I have experienced firsthand that it will get better and that ST will help.
>
> — SP/SR participant

The Vulnerable Child mode can be viewed as the aspect of our experience in which the emotions resulting from unmet core childhood needs are felt. The Vulnerable Child Mode Management Plan is the next step after recognizing your experience in this mode. In Module 16 we explore ways to meet your needs when you are in the Vulnerable Child mode and then develop a Mode Management Plan for this mode. As we have with the other Mode Management Plans, we consider the need present and the current way of meeting that need, evaluate how effective it is, and identify more effective ways of getting the need met as an adult.

Notes. When working with the Vulnerable Child mode, the focus is on the emotional aspect of experience. Young children feel loved or not, safe or not, valued or not based upon the way they are treated. In ST, limited reparenting is a powerful intervention for healing the Vulnerable Child. Initially the therapist meets the Vulnerable Child's need for connection, validation, safety, comfort, guidance, support for emotional expression, autonomy, spontaneity, play, and to feel lovable; in addition, the therapist provides healthy limits, when needed, all within the boundaries of a professional relationship. The goal is for the client to internalize the therapist so that he or she becomes part of the Good Parent aspect of the client's Healthy Adult mode. As discussed in Module 15 in the context of "The Lonely, Scared Little Child on the Street" imagery exercise, at times clients and therapists have Good Parent skills that they use for others, but

247

when it comes to their own needs, the "parent voice" is more likely to be in the Critic mode. When you are in the Vulnerable Child mode, the process of caring for yourself as you would for a young child is often one that evokes a strong reaction in clients and therapists doing self-practice work. In these exercises clients often minimize their need for care and feel embarrassed and uncomfortable when they hear "Good Parent" messages; instead, they listen to the Critic's rules. These rules consist of statements such as "Just tough it out," "Don't be a baby," "This isn't so bad—I had it much worse as a kid," "I can't believe you are crying about this," and the like. When clients are able to take in comfort and care when in the Vulnerable Child mode, it opens up emotional pain and anger as they experience how little Good Parent they received as children. For our clients with BPD, a period of mourning that includes deep sadness and anger is typically part of this process. For clients with more Healthy Adult modes, it may help to do the experiential exercises with eyes closed to allow better contact with the Child mode. You may want to do the same. We give this instruction in facilitating group SP/SR.

 EXERCISE. Messages for the Vulnerable Child Mode: Things a "Good Parent" Would Say to a Loved Child

The first exercise for the Vulnerable Child is making your own Good Parent script. To do this, make a *list of things that you think a good parent would say* to a young child he or she loved. These can be statements that you heard and would like to have heard more often, or did not hear, but needed to. In the Vulnerable Child mode we still need to hear these expressions of love, comfort, protection, and validation. Try to use "kid language"—age appropriate for a small child or adolescent depending upon the age of your Vulnerable Child, for example, "I love playing with you"; "You are such a good girl (boy)"; "I love your laugh and your hugs"; "You are so creative and special to me." If you are a parent, aunt, uncle, grandparent, friend, etc., of a small child consider how you talk to them. Try to have about 10 different statements.

EXAMPLES OF GOOD PARENT MESSAGES FOR THE VULNERABLE CHILD MODE

- **Julia's favorite message:** *I love you just the way you are.* This message serves as an antidote to the conditional love she experienced as a child.

- **Ian's favorite message:** *I will always protect you from harm.* This message is an antidote for the harshness and punishment he received as a child from his father.

- **Penny's favorite message:** *No one can be perfect, and you are very good.* This message serves as an antidote to teachers' responses when her academic achievement was less than 100%.

MY "GOOD PARENT" MESSAGES

These are the messages I would have liked to hear as a child, or to hear more often. These are the messages that I need to hear when I am in the Vulnerable Child mode today.

1.

2.

3.

4.

5.

6.

7.

8.

9.

10.

Record these statements on your phone or other recorder, paying attention to using a soft, soothing voice. Listen to the recording with eyes closed, sitting in a comfortable place where you will not be disturbed for about 10 minutes. Write about the experience in the following box.

Notes. When we use this exercise with clients, we collect all the messages generated and put them together into what we call a "Good Parent" script. We add a few messages from us as well. Clients either receive a written script from that session or record the script as the therapists read it aloud. Your assignment for this exercise is to look over or listen to the script daily during the weeks we are focusing on the Vulnerable Child mode.

A Mode Management Plan for the Vulnerable Child Mode

Actions, even more than words, are important to meet the needs of young children. The same is true for people in the Vulnerable Child mode. In this exercise we ask you to develop actions to meet the needs you have in the Vulnerable Child mode.

EXAMPLE: Ian's Vulnerable Child Mode Experience and Mode Management Plan

> **Ian's Vulnerable Child mode experience:** *My sensitivity to criticism is so intense that I react with the Bully–Attack mode at times when a simple request to do something in a different way is made by a colleague. This has led to some negative evaluations, and I feel that others avoid collaborating with me. It creates distance between my wife and me. I really need her comfort and understanding when I am in the Vulnerable Child mode, but since I look like a big bully, no one sees my need.*

IAN'S VULNERABLE CHILD MODE MANAGEMENT PLAN

What need am I aware of in the Vulnerable Child mode?	*To feel valued and loved.*
How do I usually try to get my need met?	*I act pouty, and if my wife asks, I just say I am a little down or I get kind of mad at her for not validating me or expressing love more often.*
Result	*She asks if I am angry; I say "no," and she says I look like I am, and then we get into an argument.*
What schemas and modes interfere with taking a healthy action?	*Defectiveness triggers my Self-Aggrandizer and the message: "She should be saying these things all of the time. I am wonderful and deserve adoration."*

Healthy Adult reality check:	
What are the objective facts of this situation?	My Healthy Adult can challenge both the Critic and the Self-Aggrandizer: "It is OK to ask for what I need. I do deserve love. I am just like other people, not special, in that I need to communicate as an adult to get my emotional needs met." When I do ask for reassurance, she freely gives it.
"Good Parent" action to get the need met in a healthy way	I could tell my wife what I was feeling and ask her to do some of the things that make me feel loved and valued—for example, say "I love you" or "You are the best husband for me." I can also ask her what she needs from me.
Result	She told me that she is very glad I am her husband and that she loves me and would try to tell me more often. I said the same of her and we cuddled together on the couch. I felt warm and loved and that I have worth.

 EXAMPLE: Julia's Vulnerable Child Mode Experience and Mode Management Plan

> **Julia's Vulnerable Child mode experience:** I did not get my attachment needs adequately met as a child. In the present I look for the approval and validation of attachment with clients and partners, and I am sensitive to anything I experience as rejection. When I experience feelings of loneliness and rejection, my emotional deprivation schema is activated and my Vulnerable Child mode is triggered. I thought about what "Little Julia" liked and came up with warm drinks, rocking, holding my dog, and wrapping up in a fuzzy blanket as soothing activities. Since I am single, my Vulnerable Child mode needs must be met from my own Good Parent.

JULIA'S VULNERABLE CHILD MODE MANAGEMENT PLAN

What need am I aware of in the Vulnerable Child mode?	I need comfort when I have had a difficult day or my feelings have been hurt. I need to be held and rocked and told "You will be OK."
How do I usually try to get my need met?	I binge on junk food and then feel gross and nauseous.
Result	I just feel worse—more out of control and defective.

What schemas and modes interfere with taking a healthy action?	Defectiveness/Shame schema triggers my Punitive Critic, who says, "Toughen up, you big baby."
Healthy Adult reality check:	
What are the objective facts of this situation?	Anyone needs some comfort after a bad day. It is OK to want some soothing when I am in my Vulnerable Child mode.
"Good Parent" action to get the need met in a healthy way	I can get out my fuzzy soft blanket, wrap up in it, sit in my rocking chair, and hold my dog. I can repeat my Good Parent messages. I can reassure Little Julia that she is likable and I am here to take care of her—she won't be alone. I can tell her that she will be OK, and she hasn't done anything wrong."
Result	I start to feel warm and safe; I relax and feel comforted. I feel strong and safe when I hear my Good Parent.

EXERCISE. My Vulnerable Child Mode Management Plan

This plan is something that you can continue to add to over the remainder of the SP/SR workbook and beyond. Over time, responding with compassion and your Good Parent becomes automatic.

MY VULNERABLE CHILD MODE MANAGEMENT PLAN

What need am I aware of in the Vulnerable Child mode?	
How do I usually try to get my need met?	
Result	

What schemas and modes interfere with taking a healthy action?	
Healthy Adult reality check:	
What are the objective facts of this situation?	
"Good Parent" action to get the need met in a healthy way	
Result	

From *Experiencing Schema Therapy from the Inside Out: A Self-Practice/Self-Reflection Workbook for Therapists* by Joan M. Farrell and Ida A. Shaw. Copyright © 2018 The Guilford Press. Permission to photocopy this form is granted to purchasers of this book for personal use only (see copyright page for details). Purchasers can download additional copies of this form (see the box at the end of the table of contents).

ASSIGNMENT

Use your Mode Management Plan for the next few weeks and write about this experience here.

Self-Reflective Questions

What feelings, thoughts, and/or physical sensations were you aware of in this module? Were any schemas activated? Modes triggered?

_____

_____

_____

_____

_____

_____

_____

_____

_____

_____

_____

In your work with the Innate Child modes in Modules 15 and 16, which exercises were most helpful in adding to your understanding of yourself? Which exercises were least helpful?

_____

_____

_____

_____

_____

_____

_____

_____

_____

_____

_____

_____

_____

Are there any ways in which using the mode model has changed the way you view your-self or the problem on which you have focused for the workbook? If so, how?

_____

_____

_____

_____

_____

_____

_____

_____

_____

_____

_____

_____

Is there any area of the Mode Management Plan for your Vulnerable Child mode with which you struggle? What do you think could help?

_____

_____

_____

_____

_____

_____

_____

_____

_____

_____

_____

_____

Which of the Child mode exercises do you see using with clients you are working with now? Can you think of at least one thing that you might do differently with clients in the future, having experienced this work from the inside out?

_____

_____

_____

_____

_____

_____

_____

_____

_____

_____

_____

_____

Fighting Your
Dysfunctional Critic Modes

Looking at the impact of my Critic mode even now in my life, I realize that I still need to learn to be less harsh with myself as a person. ST self-practice is the best learning experience I have had so far.
—SP/SR participant

In Module 17 you will identify and work with the type of interference that comes up as you endeavor to meet the needs of your Vulnerable Child mode when the messages, beliefs, and rules of the Dysfunctional Critic mode arise.

Notes. You worked on cognitive and behavioral pattern-breaking antidotes to combat the Critic modes in Modules 11 and 12, and here you will develop experiential antidotes. After we have created some doubt in clients regarding the value of the Critic, we move to the next step: viewing their internal Dysfunctional Critic not as themselves, but as the selective internalization of negative messages throughout childhood and/or adolescence, which can be corrected and replaced in adulthood. We demonstrate this point experientially by constructing a tangible representation of the Critic, which we refer to as an effigy. Using a tangible representation serves several therapeutic purposes. It demonstrates the theory of ST that this is an internalized negative object, *not* the patient him- or herself, and usually not completely a parent. The first step in reducing the Critic's control is the client's gaining an understanding that it is not his or her voice. Clients typically draw a face on the effigy that looks like a monster or demon. This characterization is useful, as the Critic does not even look human, underlining the point that it is the selective internalization of only the negative aspects of caregivers, not the whole persons. This awareness is not as threatening to clients' current relationships with parents or to any support or positive experiences they have had with them. It avoids the panic of abandonment that comes from the message that clients must separate from their parents or other attachment figures, losing whatever good is in those relationships. This view of the Dysfunctional Critic mode also lowers the likelihood of running into issues of family loyalty. The Dysfunctional Critic effigy evokes a lot of emotion, beginning at times with fear, but moving on to anger and hopefully rejection of its damaging messages.

 EXERCISE. Combatting Your Dysfunctional Critic's Messages

1. Write down three to five of the messages you are aware of from your Dysfunctional Critic mode. In particular, write down whatever Critic messages of which you aware that are related to your identified problem.

EXAMPLE: Penny's Dysfunctional Critic Message

- You are an *idiot—you* make mistakes.
- You *should do better.*
- You are *lazy.*
- You are *difficult.*
- You *need to work harder—you play too much.*

MY DYSFUNCTIONAL CRITIC'S MESSAGES

-
-
-
-
-

2. Now make a simple line drawing of the face of your Critic on a large piece of paper or on whiteboard. This is an exercise where being a "bad" artist is a plus, for the uglier the Critic is, all the better. Next draw a smaller face to represent the Vulnerable Child. This too should just be simple—a round face with neutral or sad eyes and mouth.

Penny's drawing of her Critic and Little Child.

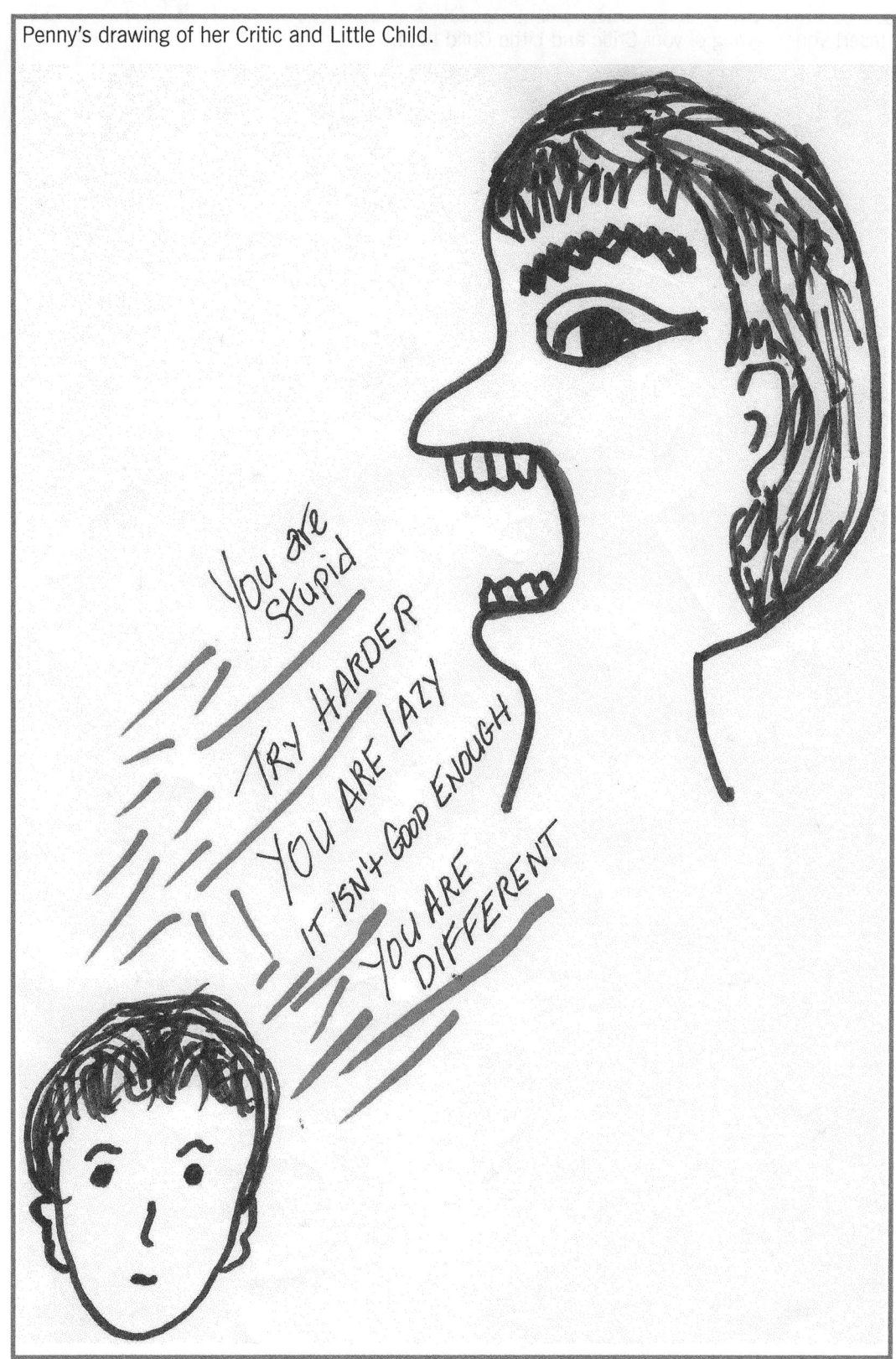

Insert your drawing of your Critic and Little Child here.

3. Now transfer the messages of your Critic onto sticky notes—one on each note.

4. Place these sticky notes over the face of your Vulnerable Child drawing.

5. Sit back and take a look at the effect. The little child is essentially smothered by these negative messages. He/she is very difficult or impossible to reach underneath this negativity. (See Penny's drawing.)

 EXERCISE. Answering the Dysfunctional Critic from the Good Parent of Your Healthy Adult

1. Remove the sticky notes from the Child figure.

2. Look at each message and rewrite it on another sticky note, changing it to what you "should have heard"—the positive statements that any little child deserved to hear.

3. For this exercise use young child-level language (e.g., "I love you just the way you are"; "You're precious to me"; I'm so glad you are my kid"; "You are a really great kid"; "I will always be here for you"; "I will protect you"). If more advanced wording comes to mind, like "I'm proud of your accomplishments," translate it into simpler wording, such as "You're just great" or "I'm happy that you're my kid."

 EXAMPLE: Penny's Rewritten Messages from Her Good Parent

You should have said:
• You are a smart little girl. Mistakes are how we learn.
• What you have done is good enough.
• You work hard and deserve some time to play.
• I love you just the way you are. You are a fun kid.
• Keep playing; it's good for you.
• I love to hear your laughter.

REWRITTEN GOOD PARENT MESSAGES TO MY LITTLE CHILD
•
•
•
•
•

-
-

4. Shred the Critic messages into tiny pieces and dispose of them however you like.

5. One at a time press the Good Parent sticky note messages onto the face of your Critic drawing, covering it up as completely as you can. With each sticky notes you place, say out loud "You should have said . . . [insert the Good Parent message here]." We deliberately use "you" language in challenging the Dysfunctional Critic mode because the challenges come from the Good Parent part of the Healthy Adult mode and are directed to the Vulnerable Child mode.

6. Take a photo of your Critic covered up by Good Parent messages.

7. Now take the Good Parent message notes off the Critic and place them around your Vulnerable Child drawing—not on the Child this time, but surrounding him or her. Get rid of the Critic by tearing it up, throwing it in a wastebasket, putting it on the floor and stomping on it, etc. Change the Child's mouth to a smile.

8. Sit back and look at the Child. What are you thinking and feeling?

9. Take a photo of the Child Mode drawing surrounded by Good Parent messages.

EXERCISE. Your Dysfunctional Critic versus Your Good Parent

Another step of this exercise is to place the Critic and Good Parent messages side by side.

 EXAMPLE: Penny's Messages

My Critic messages	My Good Parent messages
You are an idiot—you make mistakes.	You are a smart little girl. Mistakes are how we learn.
You should do better.	What you have done is good enough.
You are lazy.	You work hard and deserve some time to play.
You are difficult.	I love you just the way you are.
You need to work harder; you play too much.	Keep playing; I love to hear your laughter. You are a fun kid.

MY CRITIC AND GOOD PARENT MESSAGES	
My Critic messages	**My Good Parent messages**

As a child, you had no choice about the messages you were given, but as an adult you can make a choice about which messages you keep—and you are able to add the healthy messages you deserved to hear. Look at the table of messages you created. **Which messages are you going to give to the Vulnerable Child part of you? List them in the following box:**

Transitional Objects for the Vulnerable Child Mode

Notes. Very young children must develop object permanence (the cognitive ability to know that a parent or caretaker exists even when that person is not present) and object constancy (awareness that a relationship or connection with a parent or caretaker exists even when no need is actively being met) to cope with separation anxiety. The next step in healthy development is internalization—the ability to evoke the soothing image of a parent when he or she is not physically present. This is how the ability to self-soothe is developed. In this developmental process children have items such as blankets and stuffed animals as transitional objects that remind them of the soothing from the parent—being tucked into bed, for example, with a soft, warm blanket. Having that tangible object that represents the parent helps the young child feel the realness of the parent.

The feelings of pain, fear, loneliness, sadness, etc., that you become aware of when the Vulnerable Child mode is triggered go back to the childhood experience of not getting your needs met. We use imagery to provide experiences to your Vulnerable Child mode of needs being met. It follows that a transitional object for your Vulnerable Child mode would facilitate this process. These objects can help your Vulnerable Child mode make the transition from comfort and soothing coming from the outside (e.g., therapists, significant others) to being able to provide it from the inside—that is, from the Good Parent part of your Healthy Adult mode. This is another of the ways that ST can help correct those things that you missed as a child. To help clients recall the Good Parent script and to aid the process of internalization, we give them transitional objects in connection with this exercise. The use of transitional objects is consistent with the attention of ST to the developmental level of the Vulnerable Child mode. Transitional objects are used as an adjunct to limited reparenting. We use things such as a soft piece of fleece, with or without a scent the therapist uses; a special bead from the therapist on a piece of cord, notes with our Good Parent messages on them. The Good Parent script and other messages to the Vulnerable Child mode can be made into written or audio flashcards, poems, songs, drawings, or any other transitional object that is tangible and can be available outside of therapy. We ask clients about their use of comfort blankets, stuffed animals, etc., when they were children. They usually had something that was special to them, and many also have a story of their parent throwing it out and their feeling devastated. We tell them that just as they are developing and being able to access a "Good Parent figure" in themselves, transitional objects from us can remind them of comfort that they have experienced in imagery exercises or just from being in the safe, accepting environment of the therapy office. It is important to give the rationale for the object, thus appealing to both the Vulnerable Child mode and the Healthy Adult mode.

EXERCISE. Choosing a Transitional Object

1. Select an object for your Vulnerable Child mode that has some personal meaning for you and that you can link easily to your Good Parent messages.

2. Take it with you to a quiet place where you can be alone and recall the experience of hearing your Good Parent script.

3. Write about the experience in the following box.

Self-Reflective Questions

What feelings, thoughts, and physical sensations were you aware of during the following steps of the exercises: When covering the little child's face with negative messages? When giving those messages back to the Critic mode? When surrounding the child with Good Parent messages?

_____

_____

_____

_____

_____

_____

_____

_____

_____

_____

_____

_____

_____

_____

Which part of the exercise did you like the best or find the most helpful? Which did you like the least or find the least helpful? Which parts were the most and the least comfortable?

_____

_____

_____

_____

_____

_____

_____

_____

_____

_____

_____

_____

_____

_____

Did you find yourself thinking "This is silly" or other messages from your Critic mode? Was another mode triggered? Which one? How did you deal with any interference?

_____

_____

_____

_____

_____

_____

_____

_____

_____

_____

_____

_____

How easy was it to access critical messages from childhood or adolescence? How easy was it to rewrite the messages in terms of what you should have heard?

_____

_____

_____

_____

_____

_____

_____

_____

_____

_____

_____

_____

_____

After experiencing this exercise, can you see yourself using it with your clients? If not, what would stop you?

_____

_____

_____

_____

_____

_____

_____

_____

_____

_____

_____

_____

_____

MODULE 18

Healing Your Vulnerable Child Mode

> From the self-practice imagery rescripting experience, I can gen-
> uinely encourage clients to allow themselves to grieve losses by
> crying, as I could reassure them that they would stop. Often clients
> (and me too) fear that if they started crying, they would never stop.
> —SP/SR participant

In Module 18 we focus on experiential interventions to heal your Vulnerable Child
mode. These interventions provide corrective emotional experiences of having childhood needs met that exist today in the Vulnerable Child mode. The exercises include
imagery rescripting via written exercises with the option of recording the rescripted
scene. We suggest that you not try to rescript physical or sexual abuse trauma on your
own. This should be done with the support of a therapist. Emotional trauma, of course,
can be just as damaging—so do not choose a severely emotionally traumatic experience,
such as the death of a parent, but rather focus on a situation related to your identified
problem in which you needed a good parent, and no one was there.

Notes. Imagery rescripting is one of the main experiential interventions of ST. We
begin by giving clients a rationale for it and a basic explanation of how it works. What
follows is a summary of the rationale for clients, which in this case will prepare you to
rescript a childhood memory.

Our memories of childhood are not happening right now; rather they are images
that we have stored of perceptions, feelings, sights, sounds, and thoughts that we have
connected with childhood events. Even though they are not "real" in the sense of "happening right now," when we bring them to mind, *it can feel as if they are happening
now*, and it causes emotional pain. In imagery you can change the ending of painful
memories by creating in your own image of *what should have happened* if the protective, strong "Good Parent" you deserved had been there. Just as we all can reexperience pain and fear when negative childhood memories recur, we can also experience

comfort, protection, and care when we experience the "new ending" in imagery. The mind works like a slide projector that puts one image at a time on the screen of our awareness. In imagery rescripting, you are changing the slide you put in the projector for that particular situation. We tell clients that "this may sound like magic," but it is supported by scientific research that the effects of imagery are comparable to those of real experience with respect to psychological and brain responses (Holmes & Mathews, 2010; Arntz, 2012). Thus, imagery rescripting is an effective way for people to heal from traumatic childhood memories.

In addition, one of the most important things we take away from significant life events is *what we think it means about us* that the event happened. So if we were not protected or our feelings were criticized or dismissed, the Vulnerable Child part of us interprets that to mean things like "You are on your own—no one will protect or help you" or "You don't deserve help" or "Your feelings are wrong or bad or too much" which can translate into "You are bad or too much." As children we are not capable of understanding that the real problem is not that we are wrong in some way, the problem is that *no one is there for us.* We had the normal needs of a kid, but no one was there to meet them. We form core beliefs about ourselves, others, and life based largely on how our needs were met, or not, in childhood and adolescence, and then we don't question them—they are our reality. Over time in treatment, our clients tell us "In my head I know that I am not bad or evil; I was just a kid with normal kid needs that were not met because no one was there." However, they also tell us that they *feel like they are bad* in some way. The implicit or feeling level of experience needs to be reached and impacted for a person to feel worthy and lovable. That is the part on which we work in imagery: that you *still feel* unworthy, wrong, a failure, too needy, or whatever other messages you internalized. ST goes beyond the cognitive level of core beliefs to impact this deeper emotional level with interventions like imagery rescripting.

Our goal in imagery rescripting is to give your Vulnerable Child part a Good Parent to provide protection, comfort, nurture, love, guidance, and all those things kids need. We approach this work in small steps because we do not want you to feel overwhelmed or to reexperience bad memories again. We want to stop painful memories *before anything bad happens.* We want to rewrite the ending, so that nothing bad happens in the new imagery experience.

Experiential Work to Heal the Vulnerable Child Mode: Imagery Rescripting

In group ST, we begin by going through the steps of rescripting a therapist's memory with the group participating to brainstorm a new ending. In individual ST, we give clients an example of a situation of moderate difficulty from our childhoods that we rescripted. We include the messages we took away from the childhood experience and how these affected our schemas and modes. This approach of self-disclosure is described in detail in Farrell et al. (2014). Using self-disclosure in this way shows clients how we do imagery rescripting, reduces their apprehension, and facilitates their self-disclosures. It also demonstrates that we all have modes; it can make the therapist seem more real and genuine, thus fostering the connection with him or her.

In this workbook we give you the same instructions we give clients, and we use an example from Penny, one of our three therapists.

 EXAMPLE: Penny's Situation to Rescript

I remember a situation that happened when I was about 6 years old and in a store shopping with my mother. I think this experience is one of the roots of my Unrelenting Standards and the feeling that if I am not perfect, I am worthless. My mother was not easy for me to connect with. She was older when she had me. She prided herself on not needing to "childproof" her house, as "her children knew what they should not touch." She loved china teacups and collected them. Sometimes she would take them out, and I could look at them with her. It was near Christmas and the local department store had a special section for children only to shop in that had items that would fit a child's gift budget. The plan was for me to go in and choose gifts for my parents. I had my purse and was feeling like a "big girl," knowing how much my mother liked it when I did things for myself. She had to convince the clerk to allow me in, as the minimum age was 9. She told the clerk how responsible and well behaved I was, so the woman let me in. I saw a china teacup rather high on a shelf and decided it would be perfect for my mother. I reached up to get it, and as I brought it down, it slipped out of my hand and fell to the ground, crashing into a million pieces. The store clerk yelled at me and made me pay for it with the single dollar bill I had with me.

What do you think Penny's little child felt and what did she need?

Here is what Penny described:

> I felt ashamed and frightened, like a bad kid, that I had made a terrible mistake and embarrassed my mother. It also gave me the message that I would be all alone if I got into any trouble. My mother could see and hear what was going on from outside, but she did nothing to help or defend me. I was devastated, but didn't cry, because then I would really have felt like a baby.

Penny recognized the link of this memory to current schemas (Unrelenting Standards) and core beliefs about worth and perfection as well as her strong Demanding Critic mode.

> As I tell this memory it doesn't seem so big, but I know that it is related to my Unrelenting Standards schema and part of why I still have a big reaction today when I make even a small mistake. I may not verbalize it, but the phrase "What a stupid thing to do, you idiot!" runs through my mind. I have worked on it and I catch that reaction—which is a good example of my Punitive Critic mode's messages—but it still pops up sometimes. I know that this memory is one of the roots of my Unrelenting Standards schema and Dysfunctional Critic mode.

Notes. In individual or group ST, the therapist would construct a plan with Penny of how to rescript the situation with a "Good Parent" meeting young Penny's need for protection, acceptance for the limits of her age, and guidance to understand that no one is perfect; accidents and even mistakes happen, and we can learn from them.

Answer the following questions about Penny's experience.

1. What would a Good Parent have done differently?

2. How would you rescript Penny's memory?

3. What healthy message could Penny take away if she had experienced the rescript you wrote?

Now consider Penny's rescripted messages.

EXAMPLE: Penny's Rescript

> *Oh, Penny, honey, are you all right? Let me get you away from this broken glass. Poor dear, are you hurt anywhere? Don't worry, you are not in trouble—it was an accident. (to the shopkeeper firmly) "**Stop**—do not yell at this little girl! Can't you see that she is upset? She is a child, and you have no right to yell at her! Talk to me about this. I will be responsible for any damages." It's OK, dear, you didn't do anything wrong—it was an accident. I know that you really wanted a teacup for your mother. I think they are pretty, too. (to the shopkeeper) "Here is $2.00: $1.00 for the broken one and $1.00 for the new one you are going to bring out for this sweet little girl."*

How does your rescripted image compare to Penny's?

Did you meet little Penny's needs adequately?

Was anything missing that you would like to add?

✍ **EXERCISE.** My Imagery Rescripting

Now we ask you to rescript one of your memories that you have identified as related to a schema or mode that impacts the problem on which you are focusing in the workbook. Choose a memory that impacts you and is at a level of difficulty similar to Penny's. Do not work with a memory of sexual, physical, or emotional abuse. Find a place and a time where you will not be disturbed for 15–20 minutes. This is an exercise that will work best if you record the instructions and then play them back to do the exercise.

1. Close your eyes; be aware of your Safe-Place Image (described in Module 1) Take a moment to recall your Safe-Place Image and have ready access to it. If an uncomfortable emotion or memory is triggered, you can go to your Safe Place and continue listening or reading the example from there.

2. Let your mind go back to a time in childhood when you were in a situation in which you needed a "Good Parent," and no one was there. Just focus on whatever memory comes to mind as a time when you really needed a Good Parent to be there for you. Give yourself the time you need to be present in that memory. Be aware of how you felt and what you needed. Try to be the little child you once were.

3. Now write about your memory. Who was there, how old were you, where were you, etc.? What were your needs? How did you feel?

4. What message did you take away from that experience about yourself, your needs, and your feelings?

5. Rewrite the experience to what "should have happened," an experience in which your needs were met appropriately.

6. Turn what you have written into an image. Sit back, close your eyes, take a few deep breaths, and then let a picture of your new experience come to mind—see the place you were, how you looked, and allow the rescripted memory to be like a video clip running in your mind.

7. Find a way to remember this short video so that you will be able to replay it in the future. For example, give it a name. Penny's name was "Souvenir Store."

8. Identify a new message—the message about yourself, the world, others—that would have developed had you experienced the positive rescript you just wrote in childhood.

ASSIGNMENT

Practice your rescripted memory a few times in the next weeks by recalling the image.

---

1. What thoughts, feelings, and physical sensations are you aware of when you revisit this memory?

2. If you discover something else that you need in the Vulnerable Child mode, add it to your rescripted image.

💭 Self-Reflective Questions

What feelings were you aware of when you read Penny's memory? When you read her rescripted image?

_____

_____

_____

_____

_____

_____

_____

_____

_____

_____

_____

_____

What was it like for you to rescript her memory to provide a Good Parent?

_____

_____

_____

_____

_____

_____

_____

_____

_____

_____

_____

_____

What was it like to find a memory of yours, when you needed a Good Parent and no one was there? What was the process of rescripting your childhood memory like? What feelings were you aware of?

_____

_____

_____

_____

_____

_____

_____

_____

_____

_____

_____

_____

Did you encounter any resistance to doing the exercise? Any mode triggering? Were there any Demanding or Punitive Critic messages triggered?—for example, "This is stupid, who needs these touchy-feely exercises?" Or "What Penny experienced was no big deal—I cannot believe that it affected her that much!" If so, how did you deal with the mode involved?

_____

_____

_____

_____

_____

_____

_____

_____

_____

_____

_____

_____

_____

_____

What changed message can you take away from the rewriting you did as a result of your corrective experience in imagery?

_____

_____

_____

_____

_____

_____

_____

_____

_____

_____

_____

_____

_____

_____

Will you be more comfortable using imagery with your clients after this self-practice? Bring to mind a client who has changed at the cognitive level but is still very wedded to the Critic mode at a feeling level. How could you use the exercises of Module 18 to impact him or her?

_____

_____

_____

_____

_____

_____

_____

_____

_____

_____

_____

_____

PART VI

Maintaining and Strengthening Change

Part VI focuses on strengthening and maintaining the positive changes you have made through the SP/SR workbook. In ST, this is done by strengthening and ensuring your access to the two healthy or adaptive schema modes: the Healthy Adult mode and the Happy (or Contented) Child mode. As described in Chapter 2 and **Module 12,** the Healthy Adult mode performs all adult functions and acts to get a person's needs met in an adaptive manner. The Happy Child is the part of us that can enjoy and freely engage in play and having fun, as we did when we were children. **Module 19** provides tools for evoking and having access to the Happy Child Mode. **Module 20** focuses on strengthening and maintaining access to your Healthy Adult mode, including the Good Parent skills needed to care for the Innate Child modes.

Finding and Strengthening Your Happy Child Mode

> The exercises that were new to me—like the ones with balloons and all of the playful elements—helped me to connect with my Happy Child and the fun side of my work. I remembered why I like doing this work so much. The moments of fun can help balance some of clients' pain.
>
> —SP/SR participant

In Module 19 we discuss the other healthy or functional mode: the Happy Child mode. For this mode the main goal is to develop a plan that helps you to access the Happy Child and/or stay in it comfortably without interference from the Dysfunctional Critic. In experiential terms, the point is to engage in and enjoy play, with its exploration of likes and dislikes, and just being able to have fun.

Notes. In the Happy Child mode we feel loved, contented, connected, satisfied, fulfilled, protected, praised, worthwhile, nurtured, guided, understood, validated, self-confident, competent, appropriately autonomous or self-reliant, safe, resilient, strong, in control, adaptable, optimistic, and spontaneous. If we are in this mode, it means that our core emotional needs are currently being met. Young (Young et al., 2003) labeled this mode Contented Child, but we prefer to focus on the playful and joyous aspects of this mode, so refer to it as the Happy Child mode. Typically, our clients have not had a childhood environment that supported their being happy or playful. This may be due to neglect, an impoverished emotional environment, or even one in which achievement and work are predominant and play identified as frivolous and without purpose. These environments promote adults who do not know what they enjoy doing or do not take time for pleasure and may not have developed any hobbies or recreational activities. Play is also an opportunity to develop and explore children's creative side. Learning more about and developing the Happy Child mode will give your Healthy Adult a needed sense of play and fun. Play provides our earliest experience of connecting, negotiating, meeting, and forming friendships with others. When play is prohibited or underdeveloped, people miss out on this foundational developmental experience.

In ST, play is a powerful tool that helps abused and emotionally deprived clients break through the blocks of mistrust and fear by providing safe experiences wherein they can feel something other than emotional pain and can learn to trust. Accessing the joy of the Happy Child mode can shatter the belief that they are "all bad." Play is an enjoyable experience for both the therapist and the client because it is a safe way to attend the needs of the Vulnerable Child, the Angry Child, and the Happy Child. This is also true for therapists. We may have a gap in learning when it comes to play. The focus for us may have been on good grades, and play may not have been adequately supported and encouraged. Joan recalls that her mother reinforced her most as a child for acting "grown up." She told friends stories of Joan ordering her own lunch in a restaurant at 2 years of age. Evoking the Happy Child mode and experiencing the joy of play is a nurturing and pleasurable experience that therapists also need.

Evoking Your Happy Child Mode

Think about whom and what your Happy Child mode likes (e.g., "I like my friend Carly, who I have fun picnics with") and which activities your Happy Child mode likes (e.g., watching a funny movie like *Shrek*, jumping in a pool, dressing up for a party). Look for activities that evoke your Happy Child mode (in essence, call him or her out to play)—activities that are fun, such as playing games, watching funny movies or cartoons, engaging in favorite outdoor sports, doing things with friends, listening to certain songs, playing with your pet, etc.

 EXAMPLE: How Penny Evokes the Happy Child Mode

> I evoke my Happy Child mode by playing with my dog. He loves to play tug of war and to chase one of his many balls. I get down on the floor with him and growl back at him during tug of war and clap and praise him when he gets the ball and runs as fast as his little legs can carry him back to start again. He likes to twirl and throw the ball in the air and catch it himself also. He puts on a very amusing show, and I thoroughly enjoy the play.

✍ EXERCISE. Evoking My Happy Child Mode

How do you evoke your Happy Child mode?

1. Write down everything you can think of here.

2. Now try one of the activities on your list.

3. Write about the experience here by answering the following questions.

   Which activity did you choose?

   What feelings were you aware of?

   Where were the feelings in your body?

   Were you aware of any thoughts?

   Did you smile or laugh?

   How did smiling or laughing feel?

Notes. Revisiting positive, fun experiences in imagery may not be difficult for you, but it is usually difficult for our clients. When possible, we have our clients record the imagery exercise so that they can listen to it to facilitate the visualization. The visualization of this module is intended to be a fun activity. If you notice your Demanding Critic popping up, saying things like "You must be able to visualize it perfectly" or "Practice more—you need to get better at this!"—stop immediately and do something that *is* fun (watch TV, talk to someone, eat a piece of chocolate).

If Your Dysfunctional Critic Mode Tries to Stop the Fun

Clients may have as much difficulty engaging in fun as they do with other experiential exercises. Dysfunctional Critic modes may be triggered or Maladaptive Coping modes. When this happens, it is important to intervene to banish the Critics from this session or get around the Maladaptive Coping modes. So, Happy Child "work" can involve dealing with interfering modes as well as setting up fun. Clients with psychological difficulties often have difficulty allowing themselves to experience the Happy Child mode. Negative childhood memories may be associated. We named our inpatient Happy Child mode group with the subtitle of "Mandatory Fun" because clients repeatedly asked if they had to attend. Our group also made a sign for the door where the group was held that announced: "No Critics allowed!"

EXERCISE. Healthy Adult Messages to Replace Those of the Critic Mode

The Dysfunctional Critic modes may have negative things to say about the Happy Child mode, in which case your Happy Child Mode may need some positive feedback. If this is your experience, come up with some Healthy Adult messages to use as antidotes and list them after the following example.

 EXAMPLES: Healthy Adult Messages about the Happy Child Mode (Antidotes)

1. **Julia:** *I love your happy smile when you are playing.*

2. **Penny:** *You work enough; you need some playtime for balance.*

3. **Ian:** *Go have fun, little guy.*

Now record the Healthy Adult Antidotes you can use to replace your Critic mode.

MY HEALTHY ADULT ANTIDOTES

1.

2.

3.

4.

ASSIGNMENT

For 15–20 minutes, engage in one of the fun activities you identified that evokes your Happy Child mode. Record some notes about the experience and whether any other mode interfered.

Practice evoking any of the positive images of fun, playful, happy experiences from the Happy Child mode activities you have done. **Keep a short record of which image you used. Build up your collection of happy memories to revisit as a counterbalance to painful or troubling ones. Use your Good Parent messages, as needed, if the Critic gets in the way.**

M
T
W
TH
F
SAT
SUN

Self-Reflective Questions

Were you able to follow through on the assignment to evoke your Happy Child? What was your experience of allowing yourself to spend time doing something for fun? Were any schemas activated or modes triggered? Which ones?

_____

_____

_____

_____

_____

_____

_____

_____

_____

_____

_____

Did you find yourself thinking "This is silly" or some other message from the Critic mode? How did you deal with any interference you experienced that kept you from connecting with your Happy Child mode?

_____

_____

_____

_____

_____

_____

_____

_____

_____

_____

_____

_____

_____

Do you understand the purpose of accessing the Happy Child mode? What is it?

_____

_____

_____

_____

_____

_____

_____

_____

_____

_____

_____

_____

_____

How does your experience with the Happy Child mode affect the way you view working with your clients in this area? Are you comfortable with the idea of using play for your adult clients in ST?

_____

_____

_____

_____

_____

_____

_____

_____

_____

_____

_____

_____

_____

MODULE 20

Strengthening Your Access
to the Healthy Adult Mode

The "Walking through the Modes" exercise gave me a way to cut through
my usual long rumination when a mode is triggered. It helped me articulate and understand what is involved when I have an intense emotion.
—SP/SR participant

The exercise was useful in increasing my awareness of mode activation.
I have been able to think about my own modes, and as a result I have
been more confident in walking clients through their modes.
—SP/SR participant

Module 20 has exercises to access and strengthen your Healthy Adult mode to maintain and extend the changes that you have made in the previous modules. There
are several different approaches and exercises to use to continue behavioral pattern
breaking in the use of your Healthy Adult mode instead of defaulting to Maladaptive
Coping modes or allowing a Dysfunctional Critic mode to berate you. Four exercises are
presented for you to choose from in terms of your identified problem and what matches
your needs. The first exercise uses imagery to further connect your Vulnerable Child
mode with your Healthy Adult mode. The second exercise, called "Walking through the
Modes," is a review in which you get information about the other modes operating at a
particular time by checking in from your Healthy Adult mode and then formulating a
plan to meet the needs present. The third exercise summarizes the information that you
have gathered from using the second exercise to formulate a Healthy Adult Mode Management Plan. The fourth exercise is an ST flashcard to help you maintain your access
to your Healthy Adult mode in situations in which Dysfunctional modes are triggered.

Experiment with the exercises and reflect upon your experiences with them to
choose what is most effective for you and what fits into a regular self-care schedule.
Just like we tell our clients, continuing to use these tools will help you maintain and
strengthen your Healthy Adult mode.

🖈 *Notes.* The overarching goal of ST is to develop the Healthy Adult mode of a person so that he or she is able to respond to adult needs and get them met in an adaptive manner. Here is what that ability would look like:

1. Care for your needs when you are in the Vulnerable Child mode. This function of the Healthy Adult mode is what we refer to as the "Good Parent." From our internal Good Parent we can respond to the needs of the Vulnerable Child mode when fear, sadness, or loneliness, reflecting unmet childhood needs, are experienced.

2. From the Healthy Adult mode you can stop the action when a Maladaptive Coping mode is triggered, experience emotions in an adult manner when they arise, connect with others, and express your needs. Coping choices are made that meet your need and the reality of the adult situation rather than your defaulting to Maladaptive Coping modes such as avoidance.

3. To deal with the Angry or Impulsive/Undisciplined Child mode, the Healthy Adult mode replaces the default behavior of these Innate Child modes with appropriate and effective ways to express the underlying emotions and needs; for example, the ability to express needs in an assertive adult manner and anger in a healthy way.

4. Diminish the control of the Dysfunctional Critic modes. Get rid of the harsh internalized Punitive Critic mode by replacing it with the ability to motivate yourself in a healthy positive manner, accept your mistakes, and make retribution for them when needed. Learn to moderate the Demanding Critic mode to have realistic expectations and standards.

5. Free the Happy Child mode so that you can explore the environment to play and learn about what gives you joy in life.

In summary, in every situation there are four choices: fight, flight, freeze, or access the Healthy Adult mode.

✍ **EXERCISE.** "The Swing" Imagery to Connect the Healthy Adult and the Vulnerable Child

Instructions: Sit back, take a few deep breaths, and close your eyes. Try to let the images from this story form without forcing them.

"Imagine that you are taking a walk and pass by a beautiful park. You become aware of the scent of roses and look around in search of them. As you are scanning, you see a young child of 3 or 4 sitting on a swing trying to get it moving, but the child's legs are too short to pump effectively. You approach the child and realize that it is you. 'There you are!' you say, with affection. 'I will sit down first, and then you can sit on my lap and we will swing together.' You put a protective arm around the child and enjoy the child's giggles. You swing higher and higher, enjoying the wind blowing through your hair and the smile on the child's face mirroring yours. After swinging as long as you both want, you head home, walking hand in hand. You say to the child, 'I need your help. Sometimes I get very busy with my work or get sidetracked doing chores, but I don't want to lose connection with you. When this starts to happen, could you please say the word SWING a few times to remind me to reconnect with you?'"

From this imagery exercise "Swing" becomes the signal that your Healthy Adult mode is needed. Practice the image a few times and be aware of thinking of the signal.

ASSIGNMENT

Every day revisit the Swing image. Record your practice in the following box.

Walking through Your Modes

This is an exercise to use regularly when you become aware that a Dysfunctional mode has been triggered or as a review at the end of the day.

 EXAMPLE: Julia's Walking through My Modes

The following are questions you can use to check in—from your Healthy Adult Mode, which includes your Good Parent—with all of the modes you experienced today.

1. **My Vulnerable Child Mode**

   What am I aware of when I connect to my Vulnerable Child mode? What are my feelings, needs, thoughts, and physical sensations? If there is distress, what was the triggering situation?

   I feel sad, worthless, sense of heaviness in my belly, I need reassurance, and my thought is that I am just a lousy therapist, no matter how hard I try.

2. **My Angry Child Mode**

   What am I aware of when I connect to my Angry Child mode? What are my feelings, needs, thoughts, and physical sensations? If there is distress, what was the triggering situation?

   I feel angry that it is so hard for me; it is unfair, and no one is here to help reassure me.

3. **My Detached Self-Soother (list your Maladaptive Coping mode)**

   What am I aware of when I connect to my Detached Self Soother mode? What are my feelings, needs, thoughts, and physical sensations? If there is distress, what was the triggering situation?

   I feel a great need for comfort food and to watch TV all evening. I want to just forget about the problems I had in the session today with Jan. I need comfort and distraction.

4. **My Dysfunctional Critic Mode**

   What am I aware of when I connect to my Critic Mode? What are my feelings, needs, thoughts, and physical sensations? (Limit your Critic mode to no more than three statements. The Critic's comments are hurtful and serve no healthy purpose. As a child, you had no choice but to listen. Today you may still hear those messages, but you have your Healthy Adult perspective to limit their effects.)

   My Critic tells me that I should give up because I am hopeless and will never succeed as a schema therapist. I will never have a good relationship either, as I am overly emotional and weak. I am not good enough.

5. **My Healthy Adult Mode Management Plan:** I have checked in with all the modes I experienced today and utilized the information I derived from this awareness to make the following plans:

   - **To meet the need of my Vulnerable Child,** my Good Parent will take the following actions:

     My Good Parent will rock Little Julia in a chair and remind her that she is a wonderful little girl, and she has friends and family who value and accept her. She will also remind her that she cares about her clients and is present for them; she keeps trying and works hard.

   - **To meet the need of my Angry Child** to be heard and have his/her feelings validated, I will take the following actions:

     My Good Parent will listen to the anger and encourage Little Angry Julia to stomp her feet and complain, because it is not fair that it is so hard for her. She will also say, "Of course you are angry. It is OK to be angry."

- **Instead of allowing my Detached Self-Soother mode** to take over, I will take the following healthy action to meet my underlying needs:

  I will call one of my therapist friends who is also in the ST program and discuss the session with her. She always helps me put into healthier perspective the things that I see as catastrophes.

- **To decrease the effect of my Dysfunctional Critic mode,** I will take the following action:

  I will follow my Critic Mode Management Plan and read over the messages I wrote to my Critic in Module 11.

- **Results:**

  I talked to Jan about the troubling session and felt better when I could recognize that my Vulnerable Child was triggered today when my client said she was thinking of quitting therapy. Jan reminded me that I was this client's fourth therapist in less than a year, and that it was not a negative reflection on me. She said I handled it well; I did not get defensive or critical, just empathically confronted the client's pattern. After I talked to Jan, I made a healthy meal and rewarded myself with watching an episode of Criminal Minds on TV. Little Julia felt connected and much better also.

 EXERCISE. Walking through My Modes

1. **My Vulnerable Child Mode**

   What am I aware of when I connect to my Vulnerable Child mode? What are my feelings, needs, thoughts, and physical sensations? If there is distress, what was the triggering situation?

2. **My Angry Child Mode**

   What am I aware of when I connect to my Angry Child mode? What are my feelings, needs, thoughts, and physical sensations? If there is distress, what was the triggering situation?

3. **My** _____ **(list your Maladaptive Coping mode)**

   What am I aware of when I connect to my _____ mode? What are my feelings, needs, thoughts, and physical sensations? If there is distress, what was the triggering situation?

4. **My Dysfunctional Critic Mode**

What am I aware of when I connect to my Critic mode? What are my feelings, needs, thoughts, and physical sensations? (Limit your Critic mode to no more than three statements. The Critic's comments are hurtful and serve no healthy purpose. As a child, you had no choice but to listen. Today you may still hear those messages, but you have your Healthy Adult perspective to limit their effects.)

5. **Healthy Adult Mode Management Plan:** I have checked in with all the modes I experienced today and utilized the information I derived from this awareness to make the following plans:

- **To meet the need of my Vulnerable Child,** my Good Parent will take the following actions:

- **To meet the need of my Angry Child to** be heard and have his/her feelings validated, I will take the following actions:

- **Instead of allowing my** _____ **Coping mode to take over,** I will take the following healthy action to meet my underlying need:

- **To decrease the control of my Dysfunctional Critic mode,** I will take the following action:

ASSIGNMENT

Walk through your modes every day in the evening for the next few weeks. Record the results in the following box. Consider whether you feel that it is a helpful exercise for you to use to monitor your schema and mode activity whenever you experience negative effects in your day.

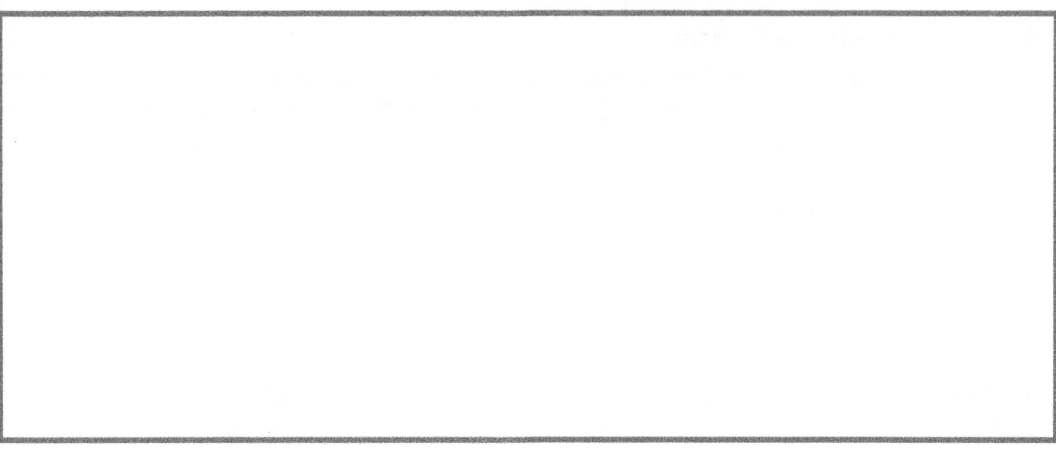

 EXERCISE. My Healthy Adult Mode Management Plan

Use the information you collected from the Walking through My Modes exercise to complete a Healthy Adult Mode Maintenance Plan. Ian's example is presented below. A blank form for you to complete is on page 299.

IAN'S HEALTHY ADULT MODE MAINTENANCE PLAN

MODE AWARENESS	Vulnerable Child mode	Maladaptive Coping mode	Dysfunctional Critic mode
Feeling	Hurt, sad	Anger, resentment	Unworthy, ashamed
Thought	I am unloved.	I'd like to hurt her back.	You don't deserve love—you are a loser.
Trigger	Wife rushed in and out to go meet a friend.	Feeling hurt	Getting negative feedback on my work
Need	To feel loved	Validation, love	Acceptance as I am
Healthy Adult Plans	1. Ask my wife when she will be home and whether I can talk to her about my day then. 2. Treat myself in a loving way—for example, put on comfy clothes, fix a warm drink, read a favorite magazine on the sofa. 3. Remind myself that whenever I am not perfect, I get frightened that no one will love or accept me, and I feel that way because that was how I felt as a child with my dad.		
Results	My wife came home early and we sat and talked about my day and what it had triggered. I told her I just needed to be held and reassured that she loved me. She did that and I felt much better. My needs were met.		

MY HEALTHY ADULT MODE MAINTENANCE PLAN

MODE AWARENESS	Vulnerable Child mode	Maladaptive Coping mode	Dysfunctional Critic mode
Feeling			
Thought			
Trigger			
Need			
Healthy Adult Plans			
Results			

From *Experiencing Schema Therapy from the Inside Out: A Self-Practice/Self-Reflection Workbook for Therapists* by Joan M. Farrell and Ida A. Shaw. Copyright © 2018 The Guilford Press. Permission to photocopy this form is granted to purchasers of this book for personal use only (see copyright page for details). Purchasers can download additional copies of this form (see the box at the end of the table of contents).

Flashcards for the Vulnerable Child Mode

 EXAMPLE: Julia's Flashcard for Her Vulnerable Child Mode

I am in my Vulnerable Child Mode now because *I am aware of intense fear. My client flipped to the Bully–Attack Mode and really yelled at me because I started our session late. My fear seems too big for the situation.*

I need *to not be there when Julia sees that client.*

My Healthy Adult mode can take good care of my Vulnerable Child mode by *keeping me out of her office and away in our Safe-Place Image when she is doing therapy.*

EXAMPLE: Ian's Flashcard for His Vulnerable Child Mode

> **I am in my Vulnerable Child mode now because** *I really let that conversation with my colleague get away from me. I said some rather extreme, negative things about him because he was 10 minutes late for our meeting. I have that feeling in my stomach that I get when I feel like I have done something wrong.*
>
> **I need** *some reassurance that I am OK even though sometimes I get a bit controlling.*
>
> **My Healthy Adult mode can take good care of my Vulnerable Child mode** *by putting the incident in context: It was not horrible, and if he seems upset with me the next time I see him, I can apologize for going too far. My reaction does not make me an awful person.*

 EXERCISE. A Flashcard for My Vulnerable Child Mode

Now it is your turn.

> **I am in my Vulnerable Child mode now because**
>
> **I need**
>
> **My Healthy Adult mode can take good care of my Vulnerable Child mode**

 EXERCISE. A Final Mode–Schema Pie Chart

As part of wrapping up your SP/SR work, complete a Mode–Schema Pie Chart for the third time. Julia's third Mode–Schema Pie Chart is on page 301. Note the changes since her first and second charts. Next, complete your Mode–Schema Pie Chart on page 302. Compare it to your first and second charts and describe the differences you observe in the Self-Reflective Questions that follow in the final section.

🗣 JULIA'S MODE–SCHEMA CHART #3

Mode labels key: VCM, Vulnerable Child; ACM, Angry Child; DPM, Detached Protector; DSS, Detached Self-Soother; DCM, Demanding Critic; HAM, Healthy Adult; HCM, Happy Child.

MY MODE–SCHEMA CHART #3

Date: _____

Divide the circle with lines based on your experience of the modes over the last 2 weeks.

Mode labels key: VCM, Vulnerable Child; ACM, Angry Child; I/UCM, Angry/Undisciplined Child; DCM, Demanding Critic; PCM, Punitive Critic; AVM, Avoidant Coping; DPM, Detached Protector; DSS, Detached Self-Soother; OCM, Overcompensating; POC, Perfectionistic Overcontroller; BAM, Bully–Attack; SAM, Self-Aggrandizer; AAP, Attention/Approval Seeking; CSM, Compliant Surrenderer; PCM, Punitive Critic; DECM, Demanding Critic; HAM, Healthy Adult; HCM, Happy Child.

Self-Reflective Questions

What was your experience like doing the exercise Walking through My Modes? Were any schemas activated or modes triggered? Did anything surprise you? How useful do you think this exercise could be as a way to regularly check in on yourself?

_____

_____

_____

_____

_____

_____

_____

_____

_____

_____

_____

How were you affected by the Swing exercise? Will you use it or another technique to remind yourself to access your Healthy Adult mode on a regular basis?

_____

_____

_____

_____

_____

_____

_____

_____

_____

_____

_____

_____

Which of the workbook exercises have been most effective in strengthening your Healthy Adult mode? What was most helpful to you in creating new behaviors and healthier messages about yourself?

_____

_____

_____

_____

_____

_____

_____

_____

_____

_____

_____

_____

How has your experience of using mode monitoring as an ongoing practice influenced how you will use this tool with clients in the future?

_____

_____

_____

_____

_____

_____

_____

_____

_____

_____

_____

_____

_____

Record the changes in your three Mode–Schema Pie Charts. How will you maintain the positive change you observe? How will you diminish the frequency of any unhealthy modes?

_____

_____

_____

_____

_____

_____

_____

_____

_____

_____

_____

_____

_____

PART VII

Summary
Self-Reflective Questions

Now that you have completed the workbook, take some time to answer the following questions and to record any other thoughts and feelings you have to summarize your process.

---

1. Overall what are the key things that you would like to remember from your experience of this workbook—the "takeaway" messages for your personal self and professional self?
   - Make a list for yourself that includes issues for additional self-reflection.
   - How are you going to consolidate this learning? What might you need to do?
   - Make a list of any points that you would like to recall when you see your next clients.

---

2. What did you learn from completing the ST Self-Conceptualization, pie charts, and the diagram? Were there any surprises? Was one more helpful for you than the others? Is there one you will use with your clients?

3. Have these exercises added to your awareness of your schemas and/or mode variants? What are the implications of your experience for your understanding of your clients' experiences? For your work with clients?

4. Which exercises were the most helpful and which were the least helpful? In what way?

5. Did you notice any cultural or religious/spiritual influences? Can you describe these and comment on how influential they might have been?

6. How does your experience "from the inside out" affect your understanding of ST? How do you understand the relationships among experiential, cognitive, and behavioral strategies and their relative effectiveness? How do you think the three can best be integrated in practice?

7. Imagery was utilized in several of the exercises. How did you experience this approach? Do you think it made a difference? If so, what kind of difference? From your knowledge of theory or research, what do you understand the value of imagery to be? Do you use it regularly in your practice?

References

Arntz, A. (1994). Treatment of borderline personality disorder: A challenge for cognitive-behavioural therapy. *Behaviour Research and Therapy, 32*(4), 419–430.

Arntz, A. (2012). Imagery rescripting as a therapeutic technique: Review of clinical trials, basic studies, and research agenda. *Journal of Experimental Psychopathology, 3*(2), 189–208.

Arntz, A., & Jacob, G. (2012). *Schema therapy in practice: An introductory guide to the schema mode approach.* Chichester, UK: Wiley–Blackwell.

Arntz, A., & van Genderen, H. (2009). *Schema therapy for borderline personality disorder.* Chichester, UK: Wiley–Blackwell.

Bach, B., Lee, C., Mortensen, E. L., & Simonsen, E. (2015). How do DSM-5 personality traits align with schema therapy constructs? *Journal of Personality Disorders, 30*(4), 502.

Baljé, A., Greeven, A., van Giezen, A., Korrelboom, K., Arntz, A., & Spinhoven, P. (2016). Group schema therapy versus group cognitive behavioral therapy for social anxiety disorder with comorbid avoidant personality disorder: Study protocol for a randomized controlled trial. *Trials, 17,* 487.

Bamelis, L. M., Evers, S., Spinhoven, P., & Arntz, A. (2014). Results of a multicenter randomized controlled trial of the clinical effectiveness of schema therapy for personality disorders. *American Journal of Psychiatry, 171*(3), 305–322.

Bamelis, L. M., Renner, F., Heidkamp, D., & Arntz, A. (2010). Extended schema mode conceptualizations for specific personality disorders: An empirical study. *Journal of Personality Disorders, 25*(1), 41–58.

Bateman, A., & Fonagy, P. (2016). *Mentalization-based treatment for personality disorders.* Oxford, UK: Oxford University Press.

Beck, J. S. (2011) *Cognitive behavior therapy* (2nd ed.): *Basics and beyond.* New York: Guilford Press

Behary, W. (2014). *Disarming the narcissist* (2nd ed.). Oakland, CA: New Harbinger.

Bennett-Levy, J., & Lee, N. K. (2014). Self-practice and self-reflection in cognitive behaviour therapy training: What factors influence trainees' engagement and experience of benefit? *Behavioural and Cognitive Psychotherapy, 42*(1), 48–64.

Bennett-Levy, J., Thwaites, R., Haarhoff, B., & Perry, H. (2015). *Experiencing CBT from the inside out: A self-practice/self-reflection workbook for therapists.* New York: Guilford Press.

Bennett-Levy, J., Turner, F., Beaty, T., Smith, M., Paterson, B., & Farmer, S. (2001). The value of self-practice of cognitive therapy techniques and self-reflection in the training of cognitive therapists. *Behavioral and Cognitive Psychotherapy, 29*(2), 203–220.

311

Bernstein, D. P., Nijman, L. I., Karos, K., Keulen-de Vos, M., de Vogel, V., & Lucker, T. P. (2012). Schema therapy for forensic patients with personality disorders: Design and preliminary findings of a multicenter randomized clinical trial in the Netherlands. *International Journal of Forensic Mental Health, 11*, 312–324.

Bronfenbrenner, U. (1970). *Two worlds of childhood: US and USSR.* New York: Simon & Schuster.

Cassidy, J., & Shaver, P. R. (Eds.). (1999). *Handbook of attachment: Theory, research, and clinical applications* (pp. 21–43). New York: Guilford Press.

Cockram, M. D., Drummond, P. D., & Lee, W. C. (2010). Role and treatment of early maladaptive schemas in Vietnam veterans with PTSD. *Clinical Psychology and Psychotherapy, 17,* 165–182.

Davis, M. L., Thwaites, R., Freeston, M. H., & Bennett-Levy, J. (2015). A measurable impact of a self-practice/self-reflection programme on the therapeutic skills of experienced cognitive-behavioural therapists. *Clinical Psychology and Psychotherapy, 22*(2), 176–184.

De Klerk, N., Abma, T. A., Bamelis, L., & Arntz, A. (2017). Schema therapy for personality disorders: A qualitative study of patients' and therapists' perspectives. *Behavioural and Cognitive Psychotherapy, 45*(1), 31–45.

Dickhaut, V., & Arntz, A. (2014). Combined group and individual schema therapy for borderline personality disorder: A pilot study. *Journal of Behavior Therapy and Experimental Psychiatry, 45*(2), 242–251.

Edwards, D., & Arntz, A. (2012). Schema therapy in historical perspective. In M. van Vreeswijk, J. Broersen, & M. Nadort (Eds.), *The Wiley–Blackwell handbook of schema therapy* (pp. 3–26). Oxford, UK: Wiley–Blackwell.

Farrand, P., Perry, J., & Linsley, S. (2010). Enhancing self-practice/self-reflection approach to cognitive behaviour training through the use of reflective blogs. *Behavioural and Cognitive Psychotherapy, 38,* 473–477.

Farrell, J. M., Reiss, N., & Shaw, I. A. (2014). *The schema therapy clinician's guide: A complete resource for building and delivering individual, group and integrated schema mode treatment programs.* Oxford, UK: Wiley–Blackwell.

Farrell, J. M., & Shaw, I. A. (1994). Emotional awareness training: A prerequisite to effective cognitive-behavioral treatment of borderline personality disorder. *Cognitive and Behavioral Practice, 1,* 71–91.

Farrell, J. M., & Shaw, I. A. (2010). *Unpublished data: SMI scores for BPD patients,* Indianapolis, IN: Schema Therapy Institute Midwest.

Farrell, J. M., & Shaw, I. A. (2012). *Group schema therapy for borderline personality disorder: A step-by-step treatment manual with patient workbook.* Oxford, UK: Wiley–Blackwell.

Farrell, J. M., & Shaw, I. A. (2016, June). *Balancing model integrity and the session limits of a changing mental health care world using the mode model, or "can schema therapy be brief?"* Paper presented at the International Society Schema Therapy biannual conference, Vienna, Austria.

Farrell, J. M., Shaw, I. A., & Webber, M. (2009). A schema-focused approach to group psychotherapy for outpatients with borderline personality disorder: A randomized controlled trial. *Journal of Behavior Therapy and Experimental Psychiatry, 40,* 317–328.

Giesen-Bloo, J., van Dyck, R., Spinhoven, P., van Tilburg, W., Dirksen, C., van Asselt, T., et al. (2006). Outpatient psychotherapy for borderline personality disorder: Randomized trial of schema-focused therapy vs. transference-focused psychotherapy. *Archives of General Psychiatry, 63,* 649–658.

Greenberg, L. S., & Safran, J. D. (1990). *Emotion in psychotherapy.* New York: Guilford Press.

Haarhoff, B. A. (2006). The importance of identifying and understanding therapist schema in cognitive therapy training and supervision. *New Zealand Journal of Psychology, 35*(3), 126–131.

Haarhoff, B. A., Thwaites, R., & Bennett-Levy, J. (2015). Engagement with self-practice/self-reflection as a professional development activity: The role of therapist beliefs. *Australian Psychologist, 50*(5), 322–328.

Hawthorne, G., Herrman, H., & Murphy, B. (2006). Interpreting the WHOQOL-BREF: Preliminary population norms and effect sizes. *Social Indicators Research, 77*(1), 37–59.

Holmes, E. A., & Mathews, A. (2010). Mental imagery in emotion and emotional disorders. *Clinical Psychology Review, 30,* 349–362.

Lane, R. D., & Schwartz, G. (1987). Levels of emotional awareness: A cognitive-developmental theory and its application to psychopathology. *American Journal of Psychiatry, 144,* 133–143.

Lobbestael, J., van Vreeswijk, M. F., & Arntz, A. (2008). An empirical test of schema mode conceptualizations in personality disorders. *Behaviour Research and Therapy, 46,* 854–860.

Lobbestael, J., van Vreeswijk, M. F., Spinhoven, P., Schouten, E., & Arntz, A. (2010). Reliability and validity of the short Schema Mode Inventory (SMI). *Behavioral and Cognitive Psychotherapy, 38,* 437–458.

Loose, C., Graf, P., & Zarbock, G. (2013). *Schematherapie mit Kindern und Jugendlichen.* Weinheim, Germany: Beltz.

Malogiannis, I. A., Arntz, A., Spyropoulou, A., Tsartsara, A., Aggeli, A., Karveli, S., et al. (2014). Schema therapy for patients with chronic depression: A single case series study. *Journal of Behavior Therapy and Experimental Psychiatry, 45,* 319–329.

Muste, E., Weertman, A., & Claassen, A. M. (2009). *Handboek Klinische Schematherapie.* Houten, The Netherlands: Bohn Stafleu van Loghum.

Nadort, M., Arntz, A., Smit, J. H., Wensing, M., Giesen-Bloo, J., Eikelenboom, M., et al. (2009). Implementation of outpatient schema therapy for borderline personality disorder with versus without crisis support by the therapist outside office hours: A randomized trial. *Behaviour Research and Therapy, 47*(11), 961–973.

Nordahl, H. M., Holthe, H., & Haugum, J. A. (2005). Early maladaptive schemas in patients with or without personality disorders: Does schema modification predict symptomatic relief? *Clinical Psychology and Psychotherapy, 12*(2), 142–149.

Perris, P., Fretwell, H., & Shaw, I. A. (2012). Therapist self-care in the context of limited reparenting. In M. van Vreeswijk, J. Broersen, & M. Nadort (Eds.), *The Wiley–Blackwell handbook of schema therapy* (pp. 473–492). Oxford, UK: Wiley–Blackwell.

Reiss, N., Lieb, K., Arntz, A., Shaw, I. A., & Farrell, J. M. (2014). Responding to the treatment challenge of patients with severe BPD: Results of three pilot studies of inpatient schema therapy. *Behavioural and Cognitive Psychotherapy, 42*(3), 355–367.

Renner, F., Arntz, A., Peeters, F. P., Lobbestael, J., & Huibers, M. J. (2016). Schema therapy for chronic depression: Results of a multiple single case series. *Journal of Behavior Therapy and Experimental Psychiatry, 51,* 66–73.

Rijkeboer, M. M., van den Berghe, H., & van den Bout, J. (2005). Stability and discriminative power of the Young Schema Questionnaire in a Dutch clinical versus non-clinical population. *Journal of Behavior Therapy and Experimental Psychiatry, 36*(2), 129–144.

Romanova, E., Galimzyanova, M., & Kasyanik, P. (2014, June). *Schema therapy for children and adolescents.* Paper presented at the International Society Schema Therapy biannual conference, Istanbul, Turkey.

Romanova, E., & Kasyanik, P. (2014, June). *An introduction to group schema therapy.* Paper presented at the International Society Schema Therapy biannual conference,i Istanbul, Turkey.

Safran, J., & Segal, Z. V. (1996). *Interpersonal process in cognitive therapy.* Lanham, MD: Rowman & Littlefield.

Shaw, I. A., Farrell, J. M., Rijkeboer, M., Huntjens, R., & Arntz, A. (2015). *An experimental case series of schema therapy for dissociative identity disorder.* Unpublished protocol, Maastricht University, The Netherlands.

Sheffield, A., & Waller, G. (2012). Clinical use of schema inventories. In M. van Vreeswijk, J. Broersen, & M. Nadort (Eds.), *The Wiley–Blackwell handbook of schema therapy* (pp. 111–124). Oxford, UK: Wiley–Blackwell.

Siegel, D. J. (1999). *The developing mind.* New York: Guilford Press.

Simone-DiFranscesco, C., Roediger, E., & Stevens, B. (2015) *Schema therapy for couples.* Oxford, UK: Wiley–Blackwell.

Simpson, S. G., Skewes, S. A., van Vreeswijk, M., & Samson, R. (2015). Commentary: Short-term group schema therapy for mixed personality disorders: An introduction to the treatment protocol. *Frontiers in Psychology, 6,* 609.

Spinhoven, J., Giesen-Bloo, J., van Dyck, R., Kooiman, K., & Arntz, A. (2007). The therapeutic alliance in schema-focused therapy and transference-focused psychotherapy for borderline personality disorder. *Journal of Consulting and Clinical Psychology, 75*(1), 104–115.

ten Napel-Schutz, M. C., Tineke, A., Bamelis, L., & Arntz, A. (2017). How to train experienced therapists in a new method: A qualitative study into therapists' views. *Clinical Psychology and Psychotherapy, 24,* 359–372

van Asselt, A. D., Dirksen, C. D., Arntz, A., Giesen-Bloo, J. H., van Dyck, R., Spinhoven, P., et al. (2008). Outpatient psychotherapy for borderline personality disorder: Cost-effectiveness of schema-focused therapy vs. transference-focused psychotherapy. *British Journal of Psychiatry, 192*(6), 450–457.

van Vreeswijk, M., Broersen, J., & Nadort, M. (Eds.). (2012). *The Wiley–Blackwell handbook of schema therapy.* Oxford, UK: Wiley–Blackwell.

Videler, A., Rossi, G., Schoevaars, M., van der Feltz-Cornelis, C., & van Alphen, S. (2014). Effects of schema group therapy in older outpatients: A proof of concept study. *International Psychogeriatrics, 26*(10), 1709–1717.

Wetzelaer, P., Farrell, J. M., Evers, S. M., Jacob, G., Lee, C., Brand, O., et al. (2014). Design of an international multicenter RCT on group schema therapy for borderline personality disorder. *BMC Psychiatry, 14,* 319.

WHOQOL Group. (1998). Development of the WHOQOL-BREF Quality of Life Assessment. *Psychological Medicine, 28*(3), 551–558.

Winnicott, D. (1953). Transitional objects and transitional phenomena. *International Journal of Psychoanalysis, 34,* 89–97.

Yalom, I. D., & Leszcz, M. (2005). *The theory and practice of group psychotherapy* (5th ed.). New York: Basic Books.

Younan, R., May, T., & Farrell, J. M. (in press). "Teaching me to parent myself": The feasibility of an inpatient group schema therapy program for complex trauma. *Behavioural and Cognitive Psychotherapy.*

Young, J. E. (1990). *Cognitive therapy for personality disorders: A schema-focused approach.* Sarasota, FL: Professional Resource Exchange.

Young, J. E. (2017). *Young Schema Questionnaire.* New York: Schema Therapy Institute. Available at *www.schematherapy.org.*

Young, J. E., Arntz, A., Atkinson, T., Lobbestael, J., Weishaar, M. E., van Vreeswijk, M. F., et al. (2007). *The Schema Mode Inventory.* New York: Schema Therapy Institute.

Young, J. E., & Klosko, J. (1993). *Reinventing your life.* New York: Penguin.

Young, J. E., Klosko, J. S., & Weishaar, M. E. (2003). *Schema therapy: A practitioner's guide.* New York: Guilford Press.

Zarbock, G., Rahn, V., Farrell, J., & Shaw, I. A. (2011). Group schema therapy: An innovative approach to treating patients with personality disorder (DVD set). Hamburg, Germany: IVAH. Available at *www.bpd-home-base.org.*

Index